The Bowen Technique

Contents

Chapter

Acknowledgements
Background History of Tom Bowen

Equine Bowen Therapy

External Factors to consider

Equine Anatomy
- The Skeletal Frame
- Hoof structure
- Muscles of the head
- Muscles of the neck
- Muscles of the shoulder and forelimb
- Muscles of the back and rib cage
- Muscles of the hindquarters

Equine Bowen Therapy Procedures

- Bottom and top stoppers

- Hamstrings

- Opening the back

- Respiratory

- Shoulders

- Head and jaw (Temporomandibular joint (TMJ))

Stretching the horse

- forms of stretching

- stretches

Useful links

Acknowledgements

I am so thankful for being privileged enough to have written this book and there is no way I could have done it without the love and support of my partner Martin Wake, my parents, step parents and siblings.

I would like to thank my very dear friend Christy Drinkwater for all of our coffee chats we had and still have on how we are going to achieve our goals and be successful. Without these chats with such a driven likeminded friend I would never have finished this book and would have just laughed off the idea like many people did when I first told them about my idea for the book.

I would like to say a huge thank you to Lotty Merry for setting up her Equine College and starting to teach Equine Bowen therapy as without you I would never have learnt about this amazing therapy let alone written a book on it! Also a massive thank you to all of Lotty's demo horses used on my course especially Neo who just brought endless laughter and fun during those long cold winter days practicing my treatment moves and stretches over and over again.

I would like to thank the visiting lecturers on my course - Julia Garrett (Bench Saddler), Toby Lee (Equine Dentist), Ali (Equine Nutrition expert), Trevor Jones (Equine Podiatrist), and Nikki Stevens (Top horse trainer, breeder, and rider). Thank you for sharing all your knowledge and helping me to expand mine.

A Massive thank you to Barry and Julie Davies who were both kind enough to volunteer their time and photographic skills to capture the fantastic photos I have been able to use in my book. Also thank you to Julie for allowing me to borrow some of her horses to use as the subjects in the photographs. They both know how much help they have given me and i am forever grateful.

Thank you to Charlotte White, my wonderful local equine dentist, who has been able to share her expansive knowledge on equine dentistry with me giving me a much better understanding to share in this book but also to use in my day to day life as an equine therapist.

To the European College of Bowen Studies (ECBS), thank you for teaching me the art of The Bowen Technique, and its use on people. Qualifying as a Bowen therapist for people was the first mile stone I achieved to allow me to progress to go to learn its use for horses at Rose Farm College of Equine Studies. I now have the knowledge to combine the effects of both horse and rider.

I would like to thank all of those people whose horses I treated for my case studies as they really helped me to understand that each horse is so different and what a huge difference just 3 treatments can make to a horses way of going and overall wellbeing!

Background History of Tom Bowen

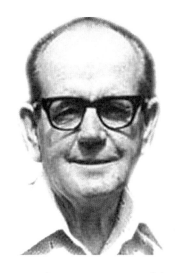

The Bowen Technique was founded by a man called Thomas Ambrose Bowen who was born in Brunswick Victoria on April 18th 1916. His parents emigrated to Australia in the early 1900's from Wolverhampton, England, and Thomas certainly embellished the Australian sporting outdoor lifestyle. As he began his working life after leaving school aged 14yrs old he seemed to come across his technique completely by accident.

Before becoming a therapist he worked as a labourer for Geelong cement works and as he developed his technique he practised on his colleges who he would treat after work, and he would also practise on racehorses and greyhounds. He had an extraordinary knack of being able to see where a person's problem or pain was stemming from and how it translated through the body.

Tom Bowen claimed to have studied many books on osteopathy and insisted that is where his technique developed from, though he had had no training or experience of body work.
He just had a natural gift for seeing patterns that emerged in the body and was able to decipher any imbalances and correct them in the most effective and appropriate way.

Tom Bowens work was reviewed by the Victorian government in 1975 when they were inquiring into Chiropractic, Osteopathy and Naturopathy. He was desperate to be recognised for his work by other chiropractors and osteopaths, but even when he had been seeing in excess of 13,000 people a year with an 80% success rate treating all of the presented conditions, the Chiropractic and Osteopaths Registration Board still turned him away in spring 1982. Even though Tom Bowen was never officially recognised for his work by chiropractors and osteopaths, he was awarded an honorary medal by the Victorian police for his services to the police department as the majority of his work was within the community and he certainly was recognised by all whom he helped.

Over the years Bowen had allowed very few men watch him work, however he did have a small number of followers whom he allowed to watch him once a week and those few that had observed his technique and way of working had been inspired and consequently went on to treat and teach people using his technique.

Tom Bowen sadly died on 27 October 1982 leaving behind his wife and 3 children who made it their duty to see his work continued.

It is with great thanks to this extraordinary man that today we are now able to treat or be treated using this remarkable technique. I think he would be presently surprised to know that his work has been successfully allowed to evolve and continue to help millions of people and animals all over the world.

Equine Bowen Therapy

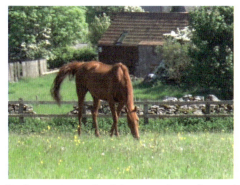

A Horse, to me, is the perfect client. A horse has no preconceived ideas about alternative therapies nor do they have the ability to disregard results and put it down to coincidence, therefore the results from treatment, speak for themselves; they either improve or they don't, it's simple. It is commonly found that most horses will need a minimum of 2 or 3 treatments to deal with specific problems they are presenting. It is then generally advised that the horse goes on a maintenance programme specific to the horses needs, ensuring the horse has a minimum of one treatment every 6 months; a 'MOT' type treatment to keep the horse correct and comfortable through its body and free of any aches and pains.

Horses can sustain quite a large amount of discomfort for a surprising length of time before they show any signs, and even then people can still misunderstand what the horse is trying to tell them and pass off the horses behaviour as 'naughty' or 'stubborn'. Because of this, the issues that horses present cannot, in most cases, be 'fixed' in one treatment; it will take a good therapist to create a suitable maintenance plan to get the horse back on the road to recovery. This may sound dramatic but if a horse has been showing signs of discomfort for 3 weeks the problem may have started 6 weeks ago or more, proving that a regular 'MOT' treatment as prevention is much more beneficial than waiting for a problem to arise.

People tend to be under the impression that because horses are big animals you need to push and prod them harder to get a reaction. THIS IS NOT TRUE! In the summer when a fly lands on a horse, its skin twitches to get rid of the fly almost instantly, this alone shows how sensitive horses are to the touch. Even to reach the deeper tissue in the horses' body the therapist needs to gently work their way in; otherwise the horse's muscles will tense up and block out the therapist and disrupt the treatment. Bowen is a gentle and calm treatment that utilises the horse's muscles and fascia to stimulate the horse's nervous system to release and realign the horses body and ensure all the horses internal systems are functioning correctly.

Equine Bowen Therapy is a non-invasive remedial treatment that works to release and realign the horses muscular structure working specific muscles and tendons within the horses' body stimulating the fascia (connective tissue) and neurological systems to promote healing, aid pain relief and conduct full body realignment. An equine Bowen therapist looks at the horses body as a whole and cannot treat specific singular problems i.e. the horse may be tight in its right shoulder but the therapist does not just treat the shoulder, they must assess and treat the whole horse as the horse may be tight in its right shoulder due to an issue in its hind quarters, ribcage or neck.

Bowen aims to release and realign the muscular structure by performing a rolling type move over specific muscles within the horse to create vibrations that stimulate the nervous system, and encourage the brain to respond by sending nervous impulses to the site where the moves were made by the therapist to release any unwanted tension, toxins or stresses in the muscle and resume normal function. So looking at the bigger picture, if you release and realign muscle throughout the whole of the horses body you are able to realign the horses entire structure. This is how Bowen can help reduce or eliminate problems such as horses not wishing to strike off on the correct canter lead because they are tight in one side of their hind quarters, and sometimes 'out' in their pelvis, and they also have a correlating tension/tightness in the diagonal shoulder which prevents them from stretching and working through their body correctly so therefore they physically find it very hard or in some cases just cannot move or perform in the way we ask of them.

Pain relief is possible through the treatment of Bowen because as the therapist releases specific muscles or areas of the horse, this releases any build up of toxins in the muscles that are causing sore spots or tension in the horse. The treatment also stimulates many systems within the horse including the endocrine system and allows the horses body to release its natural endorphins to relieve the horse from unnesseccary pain. The circulatory system is another internal system that is stimulated, effecting the horses body overall and in specific areas speeding up the rate of muscular repair, strength and flexibility for example treatment can increase the rate of recovery to an injury such as a muscle tear by increasing the blood flow which can decrease the length of time the horse is uncomfortable or in pain for.

The fascia layers within the horses body are the continuous connective tissue layers that cover ever muscle, tendon, ligament, and bone (fascia surrounding bone is called periosteum) within the horses body. This indicates that if you release any tension within the fascia in a particular area it can have an effect on other areas of the body, especially when you consider that nerves travel through the fascia in the horses body and any tension in the fascia can potentially constrict a nerve, and disrupt any messages travelling along that particular nerve. It is then to be said that by releasing the fascia you can release nerves that travel through the fascia so messages can arrive at the brain in an understandable fashion and allow the brain to send neurological messages in response. By stimulating and releasing the nervous system, Bowen has a calming effect on the horses' body and therefore helps with physical, mental and emotional stress and is able to deal with past traumas by reprogramming the horses neurological and physical memory pattern. During treatment sometimes horses can appear dazed or like they are day dreaming, this is usually a sign that the horse is remembering a past problem or the horses brain has gone into an Alfa state, a 'standby' type state if you like, to allow for the subconscious mind and neurological system to make erase or changes to the old memory patterns and reprogram if nesseccary. As we know, Bowen stimulates the internal working systems of the horse and enables the body to begin an immediate detox and improve the workings of the horse's immune system, including reducing or resolving any allergies related to things such as bedding, hay, dust and pollen. As Bowen stimulates the central nervous system it can have an effect on all of the other internal systems; respiratory, digestive, circulatory, lymphatic, reproductive, urinary, nervous, sensory and endocrine systems.

Prior to performing a treatment the therapist will need to assess the horse by making initial observations that may indicate problem areas that the horse has. The therapist should take into account the horse's confirmation and how that may effect their way of going, muscular formation, horses stance and gait, hoof structure and shoeing / trimming, general attitude and behaviour, worming, dentistry, the fitting of the tack, level of work the horse is doing, general daily routine including turn out, feeding regime and so on. It is also very interesting to observe the rider, if they are available, as they may also show signs of structural compensation that match the pattern of the horses problems, for example if the rider stands with their right hip and leg a little in front of their left hip and leg and they collapse through the lower left side of their ribcage, it is possible that they twist through their body to the left during rising trot and therefore it is possible that the horse will be sore or tight in behind their right shoulder blade and sore close to T16 of the spine as the saddle twists with the action of the rider. That is just one example a therapist may come across as any structural issue the rider has may affect the horses way of going. If both rider and horse are to be treated over a similar time period it is very important that the therapist watches the rider ride as a person's balance can be very different on their feet on the ground as they are onboard a horse sat on their pelvis. It is so important that the therapist treat the horse as a whole and the situation as a whole, therefore if the horse is showing signs of an ill fitting saddle the therapist must treat the horse and also refer the horse owner to a qualified, professional saddler to address the saddle issue. Otherwise, if the fit of the saddle is not addressed the horse will continue to get pain or discomfort in that specific area and no matter how often the horse is treated the problem will never be resolved and the horse will not be able to improve in its performance.

Commonly Presented Problems for Treatment

There are many different reasons why a horse may need treatment so here is a list of the most commonly presented issues i have come across that an equine therapist can expect.

Tight, sore or stiff in the back
Sore withers
Uneven or disunited gait/paces
Stiff laterally through the body
Canter lead problems
Lameness/Unlevelness
Tightness in the quarters
Tightness through the shoulders
Falling in/out through the shoulders
Swinging in/out through the quarters
Dangling a leg over a jump repeatedly
One sided / stiff to one way

Crossing the jaw / grinding teeth
Hollowing through transitions
Stiff through the head and neck
Muscle wastage
Change in temperament
Weak immune system
Respiratory problems
Digestive problems
Allergies
Anxiety
Bucking
Rearing
Napping
Refusing to jump
Jumping to one side
Heavy in the hand
Leaning on the bit to one side
Getting the tongue over the bit
Crossing the jaw
To improve overall performance
General maintenance
Rehabilitation

An Equine Bowen Therapist will consider all the external factors that the horse is subjected to which are discussed later in the book. The saddle and other tack, the rider and level / type of work, shoeing / trimming, worming programme, dentistry, stabling arrangement and feeding regime are just some of the things that need to be considered. After a treatment the therapist may refer you to a sadder, vet, equine dentist, farrier/ barefoot trimmer, or another therapist if it is felt necessary. The therapist may also advise you on stretches and exercises you can do with your horse to help improve your horses' way of going.

The Bowen Move

The way in which a horses muscle, tendon and so on are stimulated during a Bowen treatment is known as a Bowen 'move'; it is exactly the same for horses as it is for people, it is just applied to a different muscular structure.

Firstly the therapist uses their fingers or thumbs and applies very light pressure to draw the skin slack around to the edge of the muscle of specific area, next 'eyeball' type pressure is applied to challenge the muscle; this pressure is enough to be effective but not too much that it causes pain or damage the tissue structure . Finally the therapist will move over the top of the muscle slowly, allowing the muscle to roll underneath their fingers or thumbs. It is essential that the therapist moves over the muscle and not through it; the whole move should take approximately 5 seconds. The idea of removing the skin slack is to allow the therapist to get as close to the targeted area or muscle as possible.

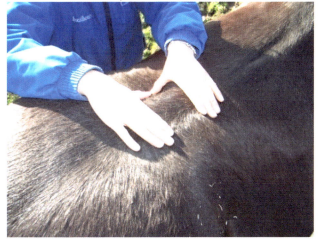

Left - the Bowen move being demonstrated, showing the typical hand position of the therapist using the pads of the thumbs to draw the skin slack and apply 'eyeball' pressure challenging the muscle before releasing.

The pause as the therapist challenges the muscle or specific area creates a pressure that stimulates the nervous system and addresses an area for release or repair. As the muscle is released by the therapists fingers the rolling action of the muscle causes vibrations that travel up the, already stimulated, nerves to the brain where the message is processed and then response is then issued.

If the horse reacts in an aggressive manor or gives any signs they are uncomfortable the therapist should make sure they are only using light pressure and use even less pressure if nesseccary. In some cases a horse may appear distressed, uncomfortable or purely unhappy with you even putting your hands close to or on a particular area of their body. In this case the therapist should back off and leave that area alone as they can come back to it later on in the treatment when the horse has settled and/or the therapist has released other areas of its body. If the horse is still not happy then the therapist could work on related areas around, above and below the area in contention or leave that particular area till the next treatment. The therapist must ensure their safety and the safety of those around them at all times when treating a horse.

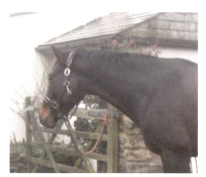 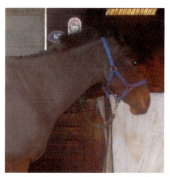

Above: first photograph the horse displaying happy behaviour. The second photograph shows a horse displaying behaviour suggesting discomfort.

A Therapist will carry out a sequence of moves and will then put in a break allowing the body to rest for approx 2 – 4 minutes. The 'break' is one of the main aspects that defines the Bowen technique and differentiates it from other therapies. The breaks provide a time period where the work the therapist has just done is allowed to take affect therefore allowing the horse's body and brain to process the information it is receiving and begin responding immediately. You can liken this method to throwing pebbles in a pond. If you through one pebble in and allow time for the ripples to reach the outsides of the pond, the ripples remain clear, complete and correct in their formation; if you through one pebble then another, then another not allowing any time for the ripples to finish then each ripple is lost and merges with another and not one ripple makes it to the outer edges of the pond. Therefore allowing these breaks during treatment allows the body and its nervous system to respond immediately and work to their full potential to gain the maximum benefits from the treatment, thus making the treatment highly effective and efficient.

The Bowen Technique is now one of the most widely used remedial treatments and is commonly used in yards across the country for a diverse range of horses and ponies. The nature of an Equine Bowen treatment is gentle and non invasive so the horse is able to relax and the horse's body can begin responding and changing immediately. The horse should feel no pain during the treatment however some areas maybe uncomfortable, tender or sore. As horses are unable to communicate verbally with people, the therapist and handler(s) dealing with the horse must always pay attention to the horses' body language and behaviour and wear suitable protective clothing such as leather riding boots, gloves sleeved tops.

If the horse is sore or tender in a particular area it may show signs of discomfort by either one or more of the following actions:

- Swishing the tail fiercely
- putting their ears back

- raising a hind leg
- striking out with a front leg
- swinging their hind quarters towards you
- kicking out with a hind leg
- cow kicking with a hind leg
- swinging the head round to bite
- biting

If the horse reacts in this way the therapist should know to back off either by stepping back for a few moments or by giving a longer break and then returning to the same area later in the treatment when the area has softened. In some cases the therapist may have to leave a particular area of the horse till the next treatment. The therapist must make sure they maintain a gentle pressure. It is hugely important that the therapist ensures that everybody around the horse during the treatment is aware of the horses' potential behaviour. For example when treating mares sometimes they can be more sensitive under and around their rib cage and their hind quarters, especially between their hind legs.

The Horses Response

Throughout a treatment the horse may continue to show signs that the treatment is taking immediate effect as the body begins to react when the muscles are released and the nervous system, lymphatic system and any other internal systems are stimulated.

The horse may show the following signs:

- Yawning – this is a sign of a release somewhere in the horses' body as the horse relaxes, it also indicates a need for a deep intake of oxygen to feed the working of internal systems. It is a very common reaction and you will sometimes notice horses stabled either side of the horse being treated will being to react and occasionally the handler too.
- Eyes glazing – if the treatment area is quiet and the horse is calm you will almost always see the horses eyes glaze over. This is a sign the horse is completely relaxed and/or has zoned out and may be reliving a past experience due to a neurological/muscle release somewhere in its body.
- Dozing – the horse may partly close its eyes and 'nod off' for a while during a treatment, this usually happens after the horses eyes have glazed over. The horses brain is now able to process and send messages round the body.
- Licking and chewing – this is a neurological release and shows that the neck and jaw muscles are relaxing and releasing.
- Gurning – the horse may open and cross its jaw, twist or turn its head and neck and make unusually facial expressions. This sometimes follows licking and chewing and normally occurs after moves have been made around the shoulder, neck and head. The horse

may then yawn, lick and chew and/or sigh. It is a sign of neurological and/or muscular release.

- Sighing – this is a sign that the horse is relaxing and muscular tension and toxins are being released. These sighs tend to either be one deep long sigh or a couple shallow breaths/sighs followed by a big sigh.
- Drinking water – the horse may take regular sips of water throughout the treatment or more often the horse will drink a large amount of water at a particular point during the treatment. The horses' body craves and needs water to remove toxins from the body and supply the rest of the bodies systems with sufficient amount of water.
- Salt lick – the horse may suddenly start licking the old salt lick it has in its stable and has barely ever touched or start licking the skin of its handler to gain an immediate intake of salt. This shows that the horse's internal systems have been stimulated and need more salt to maintain their function.
- Doing droppings/peeing – the horse may do several droppings and/or have one or more pees that are a dark and concentrated in colour and strong in smell. This is the horses bodies way of getting rid of toxins.
- Nasal discharge – the horse may have discharge from one or both nostrils after moves around the head and neck. This is quite common for horses that are stabled a lot, kept in dusty conditions or suffer from respiratory related allergies. If discharge persists for more than 2-3 days and is thick and is a dark yellowy green colour, then the person who is responsible for the horses well being should consult a vet.
- Raised veins – this is due to the increase in blood flow during the treatment. You may notice the veins become more pronounced around the tops of the legs, the head, neck and shoulder.
- Lymph stripes – the horse will appear to have vertical strips across their ribcage

- Temperature change – the horse's temperature may rise or fall during and for a few hours after treatment due to an increase or change in the circulatory system. The therapist and horse owner/groom must ensure the horse is sufficiently rugged at all times.
- Hot spots – the horse may feel hot in specific areas of their body. If an area feels hot it is usually due to an increase in activity in this area usually an increase in blood flow to boost healing to the specific area.

Horses react in a variety of ways; the above reactions are just a selection of commonly recorded reactions. If you are ever concerned about a horse's reaction or behaviour during or directly after a treatment contact a vet immediately for advice.

<u>Equine Vital Signs</u>

Whether you are the therapist treating the horse, the owner, rider or groom handling the horse you should always be aware of the horse's vital signs. If you don't already know them it is very beneficial to learn at least some of them so if the horse beings to show signs of being unwell pre, post or during a treatment and you are concerned or unsure of what to do, you can contact the vet straight away.

- Temperature should be 100°F (37.7°c). The horses temperate can vary slightly depending on the horse and the temperature.
- Horses resting heart rate should be between 30 – 40 beats per minute.
- The horses normal respiratory rate should be approximately 8 – 15 breaths per minute. The horse should be breathing quietly and the depth and frequency of the breaths should be regular.
- The horses gums should be salmon pink in colour.

- The horses eyes should be bright and clear
- The horses coat should be smooth, glossy and led flat.
- The horse should appear alert but relaxed.
- The Capillary Refill Time (CRT) should be 2 seconds (press your finger on the horses gum above the front teeth and time how long it takes for the gums to return to a salmon pink colour).
- Skin turgor – less than 1 second (pinch the skin up and see how long it takes to go back to normal). If it takes 2 or more seconds it is likely that the horse is de hydrated.

It is useful to do regular checks of things such as your horses temperature so you know what is normal for your horse.

External factors to consider

There are many external factors that affect the modern day horse that horse owners, grooms and riders need to be aware of. In today's world we ask a lot of our horses whether you are competing at the top level in your field, go hunting once or twice a week through the winter months or if you just enjoy your 2 ½ hour hacks on the weekend: Therefore it is up to us to make sure our horses stay in the best possible condition for the work required.

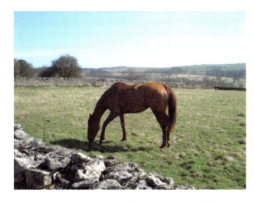

The most obvious and yet the most overlooked area of our horses daily routine would be their diet. What a horse eats and how often he is fed has a massive effect on the health and condition of the horse, the horse's appearance, the horse's performance ability, the horse's behaviour and state of mind. Horses are trickle feeders and this means they eat little and often so their stomachs are never full so they can run away from or fight danger at any given time. So often u see horses that are in very light work ie they hack out for 45 minutes twice maybe three times a week and they are on 2 large energy feeds a day because their owner doesn't understand, as they would feel guilty if they didn't feed them enough. However in actual fact they are slowly damaging there horse by feeding it too much and of the wrong things so the horse ends up either being overweight, putting stress on all its joints, circulatory and respiratory systems, or the horse gets internal problems in its digestive system, or becomes unmanageable to handle like a child that has had far too much sugar, or the horses behaviour changes for the worse and they get mood swings or become bad mannered and grumpy probably because they are uncomfortable. A Therapist should always be made aware of the horses feed patterns and any recent changes to the horses diet as this may be part of the problem that the horse is dealing with.

Another huge factor to consider for the ridden horse is saddlery. It is an area that is hugely overlooked with unqualified people regularly attempting to fit saddles to their own horse or friend's horses. It is so important that the tack used on the horse fits correctly because if it doesn't it can have huge implications on the horses way of going and general wellbeing. The bridle too can cause problems if it is too tight on the horse. Classic examples when horses become tight in the poll and generally a little grumpy are due to the headpiece or brow band being too tight around the top of the horses head and causing discomfort and pain to the surrounding area usually causing tension headaches. When the noseband is fastened up too tight, especially the use of crank nosebands on double bridles, it can cause tension and muscle cramp all the way up through the back of the jaw which not only effects the horses way of going it can also have an effect on their breathing. So often you see horses that are sore in the back and it could so easily have been prevented by having a correctly fitting saddle fitted by a qualified saddler, preferably a bench saddler as they are able to alter the saddle and adjust the flocking in a correct and effective way to suit the horse. When observing saddles on the horse, the saddler should consider the biomechanics of the horse and rider in relation to fitting a suitable saddle therefore it is generally advised that the saddler sees the rider on board the horse during a saddle fitting session. To show if a rider is sitting over to one side, sitting heavier one way or twisting through their body whilst riding, a therapist or bystander can look at the panels of the saddle and pick out differences on each side; if the back 1/3rd of the left panel is flatter or more compressed than the right the likely hood is the rider is sitting heavier to the left and this may correlate with issues the horse has through its body.

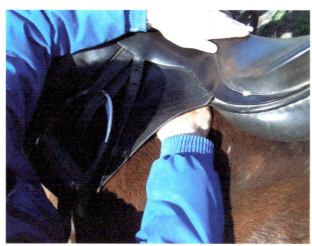

Left – checking the fit of the saddle is very important as the fit may alter as the horse changes shape i.e. when a horse comes back into ridden work after having time off whether its due to injury or holiday after a competitive season.

A Bowen therapist should have a basic understanding of saddle fitting and should always see the horse's tack, if relevant, on the first visit to treat a horse. If the therapist thinks that the saddle may not be fitting correctly or is unsure they should always refer the owner to a qualified saddler and insist that they get them out to fit the saddle correctly. Too often you hear of riding instructors fitting saddles to clients horses and it makes me want to ask the client if they would get a riding instructor to shoe there horse or do their teeth as they are equally unqualified to do that.

Always get a professional to use **their** profession to do / treat / assess your horse e.g. a saddler to fit saddles (preferably a Bench Saddler), a vet to diagnose medical problems, an equine dentist to do the horses teeth, a farrier/barefoot trimmer to shoe/trim the horses hooves, a Bowen therapist to treat the horse for muscular, internal, or behavioural problems, a riding instructor to teach you to ride, and so on and so forth.

Every horse's saddle must be checked once a year at the absolute minimum, and more importantly every time the horse significantly changes shape i.e. being brought back into work, a young horse that is still developing, or a horse that is changing its occupation i.e. a race horse to an eventer as they will now be building up and using different muscle groups.

The signs therapists and horse owners must look out for that show the horse has or has had a badly fitting saddle are as follows:

- patches of damaged white hairs around the saddle and girth area (especially the withers),
- any scars or scabs along the back or around the girth area,
- the horse may be very sensitive along their back and or around their shoulders; they may dip or move away from pressure from the hand
- The horse may show signs of discomfort around the saddle and or girth area by swishing the tail, flattening the ears back, biting or kicking.
- Looking at the saddle on the horse; does it sit level? is it too tight at the front? does it sit high enough off of the horses withers? do the saddle panels 'bridge' on the horses back?
- Turning the saddle over and looking at the panels and gullet; is the gullet wide enough? Is one panel flatter than the other? What flocking is in the panels? What is the flocking like in the panels; soft, hard, even, lumpy? Are there any sharp or foreign objects in the saddle?

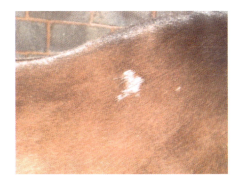

Left – white hairs on the horses back under the saddle area show the horse has had or currently has an ill fitting saddle. White hairs appear after approximately 3 months of pressure from a badly fitting saddle.

Like people, horses need their teeth checked on a regular basis, however it quite common for people to only have their horses teeth done when a problem arises. Most Dentists advice that the horse has it teeth checked a minimum of once a year, horses aged between 2 and 5 years old are done at least every 6 months if not more as there growing and changing more rapidly, and older horses that may have lost teeth or have teeth in poorer condition should also be checked every 6 months minimum.

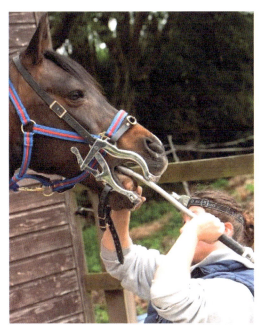

Personally, from my own experience as a horse owner and therapist, I would always advise a horse owner to get an Equine dentist to do the horses teeth not a vet, even though vets are qualified to do so. My reasoning for this is that vets only have a basic knowledge of dentistry unless they specialise, however an Equine dentist is solely specialised in this area and has a greater, more in-depth understanding about the horses' teeth and mouth structure and has a vast amount of experience as that is what they do all day, every day for work. I also think that I would always go to the dentist for my own teeth not the doctor; therefore I would always get an equine dentist to do my horses teeth not a vet. However I must stress that vets are qualified to do so.

The horses teeth can be hugely affected by the horses diet i.e. lack of forage be it hay or grass, not being able to graze from off of the floor, or a high sugar diet common with racehorses . Therapists must be aware that the horses jaw alignment can have a dramatic effect on the alignment of the rest of the horses body especially the pelvis. If the owner mentions the horse is heavier down one rein, tilts / twists its head when ridden, is too light in the hand, gets the tongue over the bit, crosses its jaw, rears up or is just very sensitive in the mouth it is likely that there is a certain amount of miss alignment of the jaw, tension / tightness in and around the jaw area and/or there is a internal problem with the teeth i.e. an mouth abscess or sharp edges on teeth etc. If the horse has not had its teeth checked for a year or more, or the therapist believes the horse has some issues they are unable to deal with the therapist should always refer on to a qualified equine dentist.

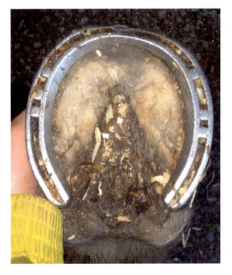

No Hoof, No Horse. This is one of the truest sayings I know! The Horses hoof is an exceedingly complex structure with many jobs so it is vital that horses' hooves are maintained in the best possible way. When I trained to become an Equine Bowen Therapist

I was introduced to the work of KC La Pierre, founder of the Institute of Applied Equine Podiatry (IAEP). I had an inspiring talk by Trevor Jones and was left realising how little I knew and how much I wanted to learn about the horses hoof, but the most important thing I think every horse owner needs to be aware of is hoof balance. Your Horses hooves must be balanced correctly, it sounds obvious but you will be surprised how many horses hooves are not, especially a shod horse as a shoe can mask the symptoms of a badly balanced hoof until it becomes a big problem that takes a lot longer to correct. The shape, balance and structure of the horse's hooves have a massive implication the structure and function of the joints and muscles above them. for example i have treated a horse with contracted, sheered heels which was very reactive and sore up through the back of its shoulders through deltoid, triceps and the surrounding area; once the horse was correctly trimmed and the sheered heels had recovered and resumed normal function the horse was no longer tight or sore through or around its shoulders. Your horse's hooves should be of even length on both the medial and lateral sides of the hoof, showing no flair, and the horses front hooves should be trimmed at approx 45° and the hind hooves at approx 45° - 55°. The horses frogs should be a healthy thick and tough, leathery texture, and the bulbs of the heels should be firm, neither spread or contracted and free from any bruising. If shod, make sure the shoe is put on straight and not skewed and that the toe clip is central to the horses hoof. There are always huge debates over whether horses should be kept barefoot or shod: My opinion is to only shoe a horse if it is nesseccary for its job ie the horse does road work every day, and that if you are to have a horse shod you should provide your farrier with a good hoof and it is the owners responsibility to make sure the horses hooves are kept in correct condition. I personally prefer to have my horses barefoot when they are not competing full time as it allows for correct 3D functioning of the hooves, which is prevented when shoes are applied. I would urge people to learn more about the functioning of their horse's hooves and understand if they choose to take off their horse's shoes and have them barefoot, they need to allow time for the horses' hooves to adjust, change and help the horse by providing the correct stimulus for good healthy hoof growth. They should also manage and monitor the changes and progress of the horses hooves over a sufficient period of time. I would also suggest that a farrier trims a horses hoof to shoe a horse and a barefoot trimmer trims to have a barefoot hoof, there is a difference. If you or the therapist is ever concerned about the horses hooves then it is always advised to either call the vet or call a farrier or barefoot trimmer for the advice.

The rider and or Level of work can have a major influence on a horses' way of going, well being and behaviour. Is it you or is it the horse? This is a great question to put forward to all horse owners and riders as many people always assume it is the horse and have their horse looked at but never consider themselves and how much of an effect a rider really has on a horse. Firstly, if the rider is present when the therapist assess and treats the horse it is very useful for the therapist to look at the riders posture as it may give a good indication of the horses way of going and can confirm or help to explain any physical issues the horse may have. Also if the horse moves or behaves differently depending on whether it is ridden or in hand can help the therapist decide whether it is a rider or horse issue. The type of work and level of work the horse is asked to do can also be a good indication of how often the horse may need treatment and the probable areas of tension combined with the age and confirmation of the horse. If you imagine the muscular make up of a typical dressage horse and compare that to the muscular make up of a typical race horse it then becomes obvious that the horse will have very different muscle configuration and therefore use themselves in a different way putting stress and strain on different areas of their bodies. For example a race horse will typically be more made up and tight through their hamstrings and a dressage horse is more likely to be more made up through their medial gluteal muscles in the hind quarters and more likely to have tension through their shoulders, upper neck and head area.

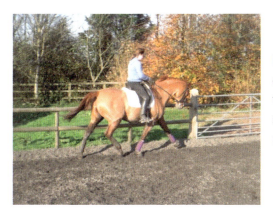

Left – Image of a dressage horse working on the flat showing his rounded muscular physic.

By taking into consideration the level and frequency of the horses work a good therapist can then advise the owner or rider on useful stretches they can do to aid the horse, some of which are in this book, and arrange a suitable maintenance plan for the horse; whether they only need to be seen once every 6 months as a MOT type treatment, or whether they need to be seen on a regular basis in accordance to a competition programme. It is also hugely beneficial and very interesting to treat both horse and rider during the same as this can really improve the horse and rider combinations performance. If the rider also has more than one horse sometimes they find a common problem with all their horses, but once they are being treated themselves they find a remarkable improvement in the way all their horses are going and behaving.

Other factors to be aware of are the age of the horse, the temperament of the horse, the horses past if known, the horses confirmation, and the knowledge of the owner, handlers and or rider. All factors must be considered to promote the horse's wellbeing and maintain the horse in the best possible condition. The horses welfare should always be top priority.

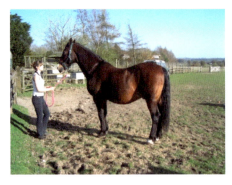

Left: 22yr old 16.2HH Gelderlander Gelding. Ex dressage horse, now ridden 5 days a week, hacked out and schooled lightly in the arena. Note the high set neck, more upright frame and slightly swayed back due to age.

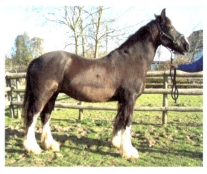

Right: 26yr old 15.1HH Mare, Cob type. Ultimate alrounder as she has had a variety of uses over the years some of which incl being a cart horse, Lower level eventer, Riding school horse incl RDA, PC, successful broodmare, and now still in full work hacking and doing dressage incl shoulder in, half pass, walk pirouette etc.

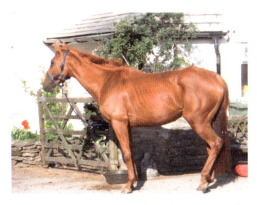

Left: 6yr old 15.2HH Thoroughbred Mare. Ex racehorse pictured 6 months after purchase (1yr after abandonment from racing). Notice the very well defined hamstrings in the hind quarters and streamline physic. She has now been retrained to be an alrounder and has competed and been placed at Novice dressage, unaffiliated SJ and Cross Country.

Equine Anatomy

The Skeletal Frame

The horses' skeletal frame is sometimes divided into two sections to separate the main body of the horse and the limbs. The axial skeleton is the main body section comprising of the skull, spine, ribcage, and the pelvis.   The Appendicular skeleton is the name for the skeletal structure of all four limbs.

Name	Function	Structure	Points of interest
Skull	To protect the brain, inner parts of the eye, inner ear, nasal passageway.	Consists of 34 bones majority of which are fused together. Mandible is the lower jaw and maxilla is the upper jaw, they are joined together as a hinge joint known as temporomandibular joint.	
Spine	Connects the head to the limbs. Contains and protects the spinal cord. Site for muscle, tendon and ligament attachments.	Large number of vertebrae , placed one behind the other, stemming from the base of the skull to the end of the dock in the tail. 7 cervical, 18 thoracic, 6 lumbar, 5 fused sacral, and an average of 15 - 18 coccygeal verabrae.	First cervical vertebrae is called the atlas allows the horse to move his head up and down and flex over at the pole when working on the bit. This is followed by the second

			cervical verabrae called the axis which allows the horse to flex it head from side to side when asking for inside or outside bend in flatwork.
Ribcage	Protects the heart and lungs.	18 pairs of ribs in total. The first 8 pairs of ribs known as the true ribs, connect directly to the sternum. The last 10 pairs of ribs known as the false ribs attach to the sternum by cartilage.	
Pelvis	Protection of the uterus.	The pelvis is made up of 3 bones – ileum, ischium and the pubis. The pelvis is joined to the spine by sacroiliac joints.	

Scapula	Attaches the forelimbs to the spine via muscles and ligaments. Absorbs the concussion travelling up through the forelimb. Allows freedom of movement both laterally and longitudally.	2 scapular blades either side of the ribcage at the front. Large, slightly triangular shaped bone headed with a semi circle of cartilage.	The horse scapula is not directly attached to the spine. The forelimbs are attached to the body by a combination of muscles that make up the thorasic sling.
Humerus	Joins the scapular blade to the forelimb	Large strong bone that joins the scapular to form the point of shoulder. It is a site for many muscle attachments.	
Ulna (Elbow)	A short bone that is fused on to the top of the radius to create the point of elbow.	Fused to provide strength and stops the foreleg from rotating.	
Radius	Long bone that connects the Humerus to the knee joint	The radius and ulna form the upper section of the foreleg.	For good conformation this bone should be significantly longer than

			the cannon bone to provide a surface for as much muscle as possible as this makes the horses legs stronger and so creates a more structurally sound horse.
Knee	Allows for movement of the foreleg.	A joint made up of 7 bones in total – 6 carpus bones and 1 pissiform bone. 3 carpus bones sit on top of the other 3 carpus bones with the pissiform bone located at the back.	The horses knee joint is the equivalent of a persons' wrist joint.
Cannon bone	Weight / load bearing bone. Joins the knee joint to the fetlock joint at the long pastern. The larger the circumference of the cannon bone the more ability the horse has to do more intense work and bear weight.	The main bone that makes up the lower foreleg. The circumference of the top of the cannon bone is what is referred to as 9" bone etc	For good conformation this bone needs to be clean from all blemishes, short and a wide circumference to be a strong, weight bearing bone. This makes for a more structurally sound horse.

Splint bones	Current function in the modern horse is to support the carpus bones in the knee. Original function was lost through evolution.	2 bones either side of each the cannon bone. Approx. 2/3rds of the cannon bone in length.	The splint bones are what the horse has left of its toes that were lost in evolution.
Sesamoid bones	2 sesamoid bones create a gulley to allow tendons to run through creating a pulley like system for the movement of the joints in the leg below.	2 sphere like bones that sit behind the fetlock joint.	
Long Pastern	Joins the fetlock joint to the pastern joint. . Site for tendon and ligament attachments	Small strong bone.	
Short pastern	Joins the long pastern at the pastern joint and joins to the pedal bone inside the hoof at the coffin joint. Site for	Smaller of the two pastern bones.	

	ligament and tendon attachments.		
Pedal bone	Site for tendon and ligament attachment.	Hoof shaped bone situated in the hoof itself.	The shape of the pedal bone is a direct relation to the shape the horses hoof should be. Bad farriery or trimming of the hoof from an early age over a long period of time can in some cases damage the shape of the pedal bone.
Navicular bone	Protects the joint from impact concussion and operates as a pulley for the deep digital flexor tendon.	Small sesamoid bone situated behind the pedal bone.	Site of naviculitus.
(Hind Leg) Femur	Joins the pelvis at the hip joint at a 115 degree angle. Allows for flexion,	Very large strong bone.	At the lower part of the femur is the biggest joint in the horses

	extension, Abduction, adduction, rotation and circumduction.		body, the stifle joint. It is a hinge joint made up from the femur, patella, and the tibia. It allows the horses leg to swing backwards and forwards.
Patella	Locks the horses legs when the horses is dosing by hooking the patella over the inner trochlear ridge of the femur.	A form of sesamoid bone situated in the stifle joint.	Similar to a persons' knee cap.
Tibia	Forms the upper part of the hind leg. Connects the stifle joint to the hock.	Large bone situated between the femur and the tarsal bones of the hock.	
Fibula	Fused to the top of the tibia to form the upper part of the hind leg and provide extra strength.	Smaller bone fused to the top of the tibia. It extends half the length and sits parallel to the tibia on the caudal lateral side (back, outside edge of tibia).	

Tarsal bones (hock)	Hock is used for shock absorption to limit concussion.	6 bones in total set out in 3 rows. There are 5 tarsus bones and 1 calcaneus bone situated at the back forming he point of hock.	Where the tibia meets the talus (tibial tarsal) and calcaneus (Fibular tarsal) is known as the tibiotarsal joint. This hinge joint can perform flexion and extension.
Cannon bone	Weight / load bearing bone. Joins the hock at the tarsometatarsal joint to the fetlock joint at the long pastern.	Main Bone that makes up the lower part of the Hind leg. The hind cannon bones are longer than those of the foreleg.	
Splint bones	Current function in the modern horse is to support the tarsus bones in the hock. Original function was lost through evolution.	2 bones either side of each the cannon bone. Approx. 2/3rds of the cannon bone in length.	The splint bones are what the horse has left of its toes that were lost in evolution.
Sesamoid bones	2 sesamoid bones create a gulley to allow tendons to run through	2 Sphere like bones that sit behind the fetlock joint.	

	creating a pulley like system for the movement of the joints in the leg below.		
Long pastern	Joins the fetlock joint to the pastern joint. Site for tendon and ligament attachments.	Small strong bone situated between the cannon bone and short pastern.	
Short pastern	Joins the long pastern at the pastern joint and joins to the pedal bone inside the hoof at the coffin joint. Site for ligament and tendon attachments.	Smaller of the 2 pastern bones.	
Pedal bone	Site for tendon and ligament attachment.	Hoof shaped bone situated in the hoof itself.	The shape of the pedal bone is a direct relation to the shape the horses hoof should be. Bad farriery or trimming of the hoof from an early age over a long period of time

			can in some cases damage the shape of the pedal bone.
Navicular bone	Protects the joint and tendons from concussion and pressure.	Small sesamoid bone situated behind the pedal bone.	Site of Navicular disease – potentially due to the inflammation of the Navicular synovial bursa between the Navicular bone and the deep flexor tendon.

The horses skeletal frame

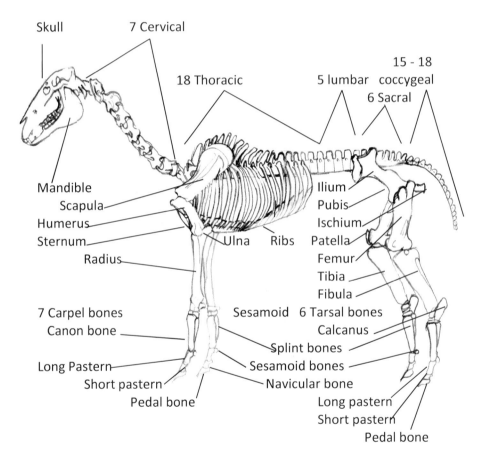

The foreleg   The Hind leg

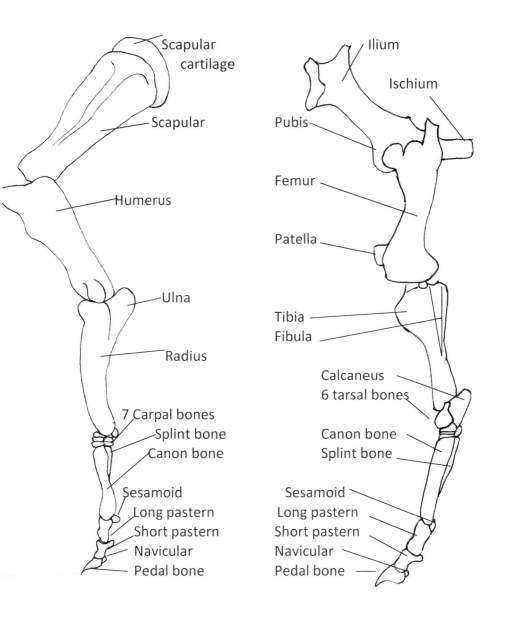

Anatomy of the horses hoof

Name	Function	Structure	Points of interest
Hoof wall	Protects the internal structure and workings of the hoof	Horny layer that extends down from the coronary band.	
Coronet band	Production of Periople. Acts as a pump regulating blood flow in and out of the hoof.	Soft white band around the top of the hoof.	The contracting and expanding of the coronet band as the horses hoof lands and retracts from the floor is the main regulator of the blood flow pressure in and out of the horse's hooves.
Periople	Protects and prevents the new hoof wall from being damaged and protects the rest of the outside of the hoof wall. It also helps to protect the coronary band from becoming bruised from shock	A transparent layer that covers the area of newly formed hoof wall just below the coronary band and then thins out and spans over the hoof wall surface.	

	absorption coming up through the hoof wall.		
Inner hoof wall (lamina)	Provides protection to the inner structure of the hoof. Allows for 3D movement of the hoof.	Pale Cream / white intertubular horn that binds tubules together. Not to be mistaken for the 'white line'.	There is a higher ratio of moisture in the inner hoof wall in comparison to the outer hoof wall allowing the inner hoof wall to be more pliable and able to stretch with the movement of the outer hoof wall. Having the hoof wall separated into 2 different sections also allows the internal structure of the hoof to be better protected against shock absorption.
White Line	Acts as a solvent joining the inner hoof wall to the sole. Creates a barrier against bacterial infiltration	Pale yellowy substance between the sole and the hoof wall.	Actually a pale yellowy golden colour and not white as the name suggests. This creates a shallow groove around the

			base of the hoof made to collect dirt to aid with traction.
Sole	Provides protection for the inner workings of the hoof. Outer sole also acts as a weight baring surface to aid the hoof wall.	Underside of the hoof contained inside the white line, not including the frog and bars.	
Frog	It provides a resistance to distortion of the hoof capsule during the stride.	A wide and substantial triangular shape, made of a thick, tough, leathery material.	On contra to most people's belief the frog is not the sole 'pump' for the circulation for the horses hoof and lower limb.
Bars	Controls the movement of the back of the hoof, adding to the strength of the heels.	Continuation of the hoof wall on the underside of the hoof wall either side of the frog.	
Collateral groove	Allows for 3D movement of the Hoof to effectively absorb concussion.	Groove between the wall of the bar and sole, and the wall of the frog.	

Heel bulbs	Protects the lateral cartilages, absorbs shock and resists distortion of the hoof.	Thick fatty area joining the horses frog to the outer hoof wall and the tissues and skin at the back of the short pastern.	
Internal structure Short Pastern bone	Joins the long pastern at the pastern joint and joins to the pedal bone inside the hoof at the coffin joint. Site for ligament and tendon attachments.	Smaller of the 2 pastern bones	
Pedal Bone	Site for tendon and ligament attachment	Hoof shaped bone situated in the hoof itself.	The shape of the pedal bone is a direct relation to the shape the horses hoof should be. Bad farriery or trimming of the hoof from an early age over a long period of time can in some cases damage the shape of the pedal bone.

Navicular bone	Protects the joint and tendons from concussion and pressure.	Small sesamoid bone situated behind the pedal bone	Site of Navicular disease – potentially due to the inflammation of the Navicular synovial bursa between the Navicular bone and the deep flexor tendon.
Digital cushion	Absorbs shock through blood transfer.	Situated behind the pedal bone and above the frog.	The health of the digital cushion has a direct effect on the pedal bone and any inflammation of the digital cushion can distort the angle of the pedal bone.
Lateral cartilage	Absorb shock and act as a spring releasing energy during active motion; they suspend the pedal bone and prevent the decent of the pedal bone during weight bearing situations such as landing after a jump.	They are easiest found at the back of the hoof spreading both above and below the coronary band and extending from the back around the sides and front of the hoof. The lower part of the lateral cartilages spreads over	The lateral cartilages also form a matrix that goes under the digital cushion supporting it like a sling.

		the digital cushion and attaches to the back of the pedal bone.	
Venous Plexuses	Supplies a plentiful amount of blood to nourish and aid the workings of each of the horse's hooves.	Assembly of five veins inside each one of the horses hooves.	Solar plexus nourishes the horn which creates the corium that generates the sole. Digital Plexus supplies the digital cushion with blood. Lateral Plexus supplies the lateral cartilages with blood. Lamellae plexus supplies blood to nourish the corium that creates the intertubular inner hoof wall. Coronary plexus supplies nutrients in the blood to the coronary band corium that produces the tubules inside the hoof wall.

Anatomy of the hoof

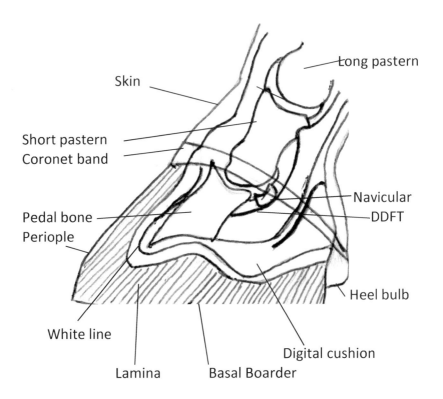

Muscular Frame

Muscles of the Head

The muscles, tendons and ligaments that make up the horses head are sometimes widely overlooked and in some cases where the horse is tight in a particular point on its head it can cause large imbalances in the rest of the horses body. It is important that a horse has their teeth looked at a minimum of once a year as a problem with a tooth on one side of the horse's mouth can not only cause digestive issues it can change the way the horses muscles work in the horses head. It is also important to remember that the muscular structure of the head is complex and one area can have a direct impact on another, for example, horses that have been unkindly twitched by their ears may be tight in under the jaw which can cause tension all down the underside of their necks and into their chest potentially causing the horse to have short or choppy striding. Like humans, horses can suffer from headaches due to tension through the muscles around the head. This is usually caused by one of three thing; stress – if the horse feels under excess pressure or in an environment they are not comfortable with, Dehydration – if the horse is not drinking enough water to remove toxins from the muscles in the body, or an ill fitting bridle/ halter / headcollar – if the brow band, noseband or headpiece is too tight it can case unnesseccary pressure on the horses head.

Name	Function	Structure	Points of interest
Massater	Aids chewing, joins the mandible and maxilla	Large flat sheet like muscle.	
Zygomaticus (Retractor muscle of angle of mouth)	Lifts and moves the corner of the mouth, aids chewing and movement of the lips.	Long cylinder type muscle running fron the corner of the mouth to half way along the facial crest.	
Buccinator muscle .	Aids chewing and movement of the lips including lifting the corner of the mouth.	Circular muscle	
Depressor labii mandibularis (Depressor muscle of lower lip)	Moves the mandible (lower jaw).	Strong central flat muscle	
Orbicularis oris of lips (Sphincter mouth muscle)	Aids movement of the lips for eating, drinking, foraging and facial expressions.	Semicircular muscle above and around the corner of the mouth.	

Levator labii maxillaries (Levator muscle of upper lip)	Aids movement of the upper lip	Long strap like muscle.	
levator nasolabialis (Levator muscle of upper lip and nostril)	Move the upper jaw when chewing and aid nostril movement.	Long strap like muscle branching to the nostrils and upper lip.	
Canine muscle (lateral dilator muscle of nostril)	Expands and contracts the nostrils for breathing and facial expression	Large flat muscle spanning the lateral edge of the nostril thinning down in a triangular shape towards the facial crest.	
Dilator naris apicalis (transverse nasal muscle)	Aids the movement of the nostrils	Small flat muscle lying across the front of the nasal passage just above the nostrils.	Nasal strips used on ompetition horses relax this muscle to widen the nasal passage to increase airflow.
Orbicularis oculi of eyelid (sphincter muscle of palpebral fissure)	Aids movement of the other muscles surrounding	Strong complete circular muscle surrounding the eye socket.	Above – levator muscle of medial angle of eye.

	the eye used to protect the eye from foreign bodies and bright lighting.		Below – depressor muscle of lower eyelid.
Interscutular muscle	Aids movement of the ears and when contracted gives an alert expression.	Small padded muscles rostral of the ears.	Tight fitting brow band can damage this muscle. Can get tight due to stress and cause minor or constant headaches.
Frontoscutular muscle	Aids movement of the ears when detecting sounds and used in facial expressions.	2 small strip muscles laterally rostral of the ears.	Used for moving the horses ears from pointing forward to the side and back.
Interscutular muscle	Aids movement of the ears forwards and assists in facial expression.	Small wide muscle located at the base in front of the ear.	Tight fitting brow band can damage this muscle.
Parotidoauricular (depressor muscle of pinna)	Aids rotational movement of the ear. Assists in	Thin strap muscle attaching from the lateral base of the ear	When this muscle is tight it prevents the horse from

	lateral flexion and movement of the mandible.	and behind the caudal dorsal ridge of the mandible.	flexing its head to the opposite side.
Cervicoauriculars (long levator and abductor muscle of pinna)	Aids the movement of the ear.	Arch shaped thin muscle running the circumference of the caudal base of the ear.	Tight fitting head piece can damage this muscle

Muscles of the neck

Name	Function	Structure	Points of interest
Nuchal ligament	Aids in lifting the head and neck up pulling them back toward the horses body .	Long strong strap muscle from the pole to the withers	Continues through the back along the spine as the supraspinous ligament
Splenius	Aids side to side neck movement in the cranial half of the neck and helps lift the head up when it contracts.	Large sheet muscle attachments from the Nucheal ligament at the poll, the cervical spine C3 – C5 branching to the thoracic spine T3 – T5 and caudal base of the Nucheal ligament.	Tension in this muscle can have an effect on the horses balance and shape / scope over a fence as the horse doesn't have full stretch and freedom of movement through their neck.
Rhomboideus cervicis (cervical part of the rhomboid muscle)	Raises the neck dorsally from the base of the neck and aids the movement	Large expansive muscle originating from the Nucheal / supraspinous ligament and	Can become damaged by an ill fitting saddle being too tight around and shoulder or a saddle that is

	of scapular cranially.	inserts under the trapezius muscle to the medial edge of the scapular cartilage.	too wide o dropped in front pushing in behind the scapular.
Trapezius cervicis (cervical part of trapezius muscle)	Raises the cranial edge of the scapular dorsally and forward.	1 flat sheet muscle split into 2 sections – cervical and thoracic. Cervical section appears as a triangular shape originating from the cervical spine and attaching along the Nucheal / suprsinous ligament and the scapular spine into the thoracic section of the trapezius.	Well developed in horses that work up through their shoulders.
Serratus ventralis cervicis(cervical part of ventral serrate muscles)	Raises the cranial side of the scapular dorsally .	Strong thick compact muscle originating fron the cervical spine C4 and C5,	Antagonist to Serratus thoracic.

		inserting to the medial side of the scapular.	
Omotransversarius (omotransverse muscle)	Aids in raising the cranial side of the scapular forward and dorsally aiding the movement of the forelimb forward.	Thick strap like muscle that originates from the cervical spine – atlas(C2), C3 and C4 inserting in to the Humerus at the point of the shoulder.	The muscle travels down the along the dorsal side of the braciocephalic into the point of the shoulder where it also attaches to the trapezius.
Bracheocephalic muscle	To move the head up and down.	Very Strong strap like muscle divided into two sections – Cleidomastoid section (front half of the muscle nearer the horses head) and the Cleidobrachial section that attaches to the sternum .	This muscle is over developed in ewe necked horses ususlly due to incorrect schooling.
Sternocephalic (Sternomandibular muscle)	Aiding the movement of the neck down and lateral neck flexion.	Large strap like muscle originating from the sternum cartilage and	

		inserting into the cranial edge of the mandible.	
Sternohyoid muscle and Sternothyroid muscle	Aids movement of the neck downwards and lateral neck flexion	Large strap muscles originating on the sternum cartilage inserting to the caudal side of the larynx lamina and the hyoid bones.	Lies over the top of omohyoid muscle. Can be affected if horse has bad teeth / jaw problems or if the horse has been tongue tied / twitched.

Muscles of the Shoulder and forelimb

Name	Function	Structure	Points of interest
Thorasic Trapezius (thoracic part of trapezius)	Retracts the top of the scapular back towards the trunk of the horses body.	Large, relatively flat triangular muscle	Makes up the other half of the Trapezius muscle. Very important muscle for jumping and extension paces. Can be damaged by ill fitting saddles.
Subclavius (cranial part of deep pectoral muscle)	Allows for movement and limits excess lateral movement of the shoulder.	Thick, very strong cylinder muscle that runs under the scapular at the front following the angle of the scapular.	Acts as part of the thoracic sling to keep the shoulder attached to the horses body due to no collar bone.
Descending superficial pectoral (Cranial superficial pectoral)	Helps to move the foreleg forward and medially. Also aids in stabilising the shoulder joint.	Large muscle that originates on the sternum and inserts on to the crest of the Humerus and the deltoid tuberosity.	
Deltoid	Aids the lateral movement of the shoulder and restricts	Strong, cylinder type muscle originating at	

	excess medial movement of the shoulder.	ulna and inserting to the top of the scapular.	
Triceps	Pull the forearm back during movement.	3 tricep muscles – long head, medial head and short head (top to bottom)	
Brachial muscle (Biceps)	Extend the forearm.	Small thick 'chicken breast' type muscle.	Very important for tucking the front legs up over a fence.
Radial carpal extensor muscle	Extends the forearm	Large thick muscle positioned cranially of the radius.	Continues as a tendon
Comman digital extensor muscle	Extends the forearm and aids lateral movement of the forearm.	Large thick muscle extending the length of the radius situated laterally.	Continues as a tendon
Lateral digital extensor muscle and tendon.	Extends the forearm and aids lateral movement of the forearm. Tendon aids the extension of the carpal, pastern and coffin joints.	Large thick muscle extending the length of the radius situated laterally beneath the common digital extensor muscle. continuing as a	Continues as a tendon

		tendon attaching to the lateral edge of the pedal bone.	
Lateral ulna muscle and tendon.	Flexes the fore leg and the knee caudally and aids lateral movement.	Large broad muscle situated on the lateral caudal side of the radius and continues as a tendon that splits into two over the accessory carpel bone and attaches at the splint bones.	Continues as 2 tendons, long and short.
Deep digital flexor muscle and tendon	Flexes all the joints in the foreleg caudally.	Large thick 3 headed muscle originating from the Humerus, top of the radius and top of the ulna joining together behind the carpus and continuing as one tendon that runs superficial of the Suspensory ligament but deeper than	

		the superficial digital flexor tendon and attaches to the pedal bone.	
Oblique carpal 0extensor muscle and tendon	Extends the foreleg by pulling the radius forward	Strap muscle travelling diagonally, medially across the radius caudally and continues as a tendon attaching to the medial splint bone.	
Radial carpal flexor muscle	Pulls the foreleg cranially.	Large broad muscle located cranially and covering the length of the radius.	Only flexor muscle found cranially on the foreleg.
Ulna carpal flexor muscle	Flexes the knee and foreleg caudally and aids movement medially.	Large muscle stemming the length of the ulna and radius on the caudal, medial side.	
Radial carpal extensor tendon (RCET)	Extends the knee forward.	Tendon attaching to the upper dorsal section of the cannon bone.	

Common digital extensor tendon (CDET)	Pulls upward to extend the carpal, pastern, and coffin joints.	Very long tendon positioned dorsally along the lower foreleg attaching to the dorsal edge of the pedal bone.	If a horse has damaged this extensor tendon they may not appear lame as the other extensor tendons will compensate for any weakness in the CDET.
Superficial digital flexor muscle and tendon (SDFT)	Flexes the lower limb at the elbow, knee, fetlock and pastern joints.	Originated on the Humerus and the back of the radius, and travels down the back of the leg behind the cannon bone below the fetlock and attaches distally to the long pastern and the short pastern.	Most commonly damaged lower leg tendon.
Suspensory ligament	Supports the fetlock joint and prevents over extension of the joint.	Tendon travels down between the splint bones then separates into 2 branches attaching to the sesamoid bones at the back of the fetlock joint	

		and then continues down and attaches to the extensor tendons.	
Extensor retinacula	Holds the extensor tendons in place	Loops of deep fascia	
Flexor retinacula	Holds flexor tendons in place	Band of deep fascia	Completes the carpus and tarsus canals for the deep digital flexor tendons.

Muscles of the back and ribcage

Name	Function	Structure	Points of interest
Thoracic Trapezius	Thoracic section of the trapezius that aids caudal movement of the head of the scapula .	Large flat triangular shaped muscle.	This muscle can become damaged by ill fitting saddles.
Latissimus Dorsi	Aids movement of the shoulder and the foreleg flexing the shoulder joint between the Humerus and the scapular, and aids movement through the back and supports the spine.	Large triangular shape muscle stemming the length of the scapular inserting at the Humerus and originating from the supraspinous ligament and the thoracolumbar fascia	This muscle can become damaged by ill fitting saddles.
Longissimus dorsi	Aids independent lateral movement of the spine when turning on circles and bending through the body. Also aiding	Long muscle either side of the spine originating at the pelvis on the lumbar dorsal fascia and inserting on to the cervical vertebrae, also attaching to the caudal dorsal sides of the	Runs the length of the back. This is the area that the rider sits on. Can be restricted and damaged

	longitudinal movement through the back, contracting to shorten the back and relaxing to allow for a stretch over the back.	ribcage.	by badly fitting saddles.
Thoracic ventral serrate	Draws the scapular caudally so aids in movement of the foreleg.	Large sheet of muscle that originates laterally across the first 9 ribs and inserts into the back o the scapula.	
External intercostals muscles	Supports the ribcage and aids movement during exhalation.	Superficial flat, thin muscles that lie in the spaces between ribs.	
External abdominal obliques	Aids movement of the trunk of the horses body laterally and longitudinally. Contraction aid mares when giving birth, aids horses when passing droppings and urine and also aids respiration.	Originates laterally over the ribcage approx ribs 4 – 18 and the thoracolumbar fascia and inserts into the pelvis and the inguinal ligament.	

Caudal dorsal serrate muscles	Supports the ribcage and the back and aids in movement of the trunk.	Flat sheet muscle attaching dorsally to the ribcage at ribs 10 – 18 and originating from the dorsal lumbar fascia.	
Deep pectoral muscle	Aids the Adduction of the forelimb.	Large deep muscle originating from the caudal side of the sternum and inserts onto the Humerus.	
Rectus abdominus	Assists in the movement of the ribcage and trunk of the horse's body. Flexes the lumbar region of the spine including the lumbosacral joint.	Attaches to and originates from the edge of the costal cartilages of the ribs, approximately ribs 4 – 9/10, attaching to intercostals muscles and the intertransversales Lumborum muscles and inserts onto the head of the femur.	
Supraspinous ligament	Supports the spine and flexes the spine longitudally and laterally.	Long strong strap muscle the becomes the supraspinous ligament from the Nucheal ligament at the withers and continues along the spine to the tail.	

Muscles of the Hind Quarters

Name	Function	Structure	Points of interest
Medial gluteal muscle.	Aids the abduction of the hind leg and movement of the pelvis extending the hip.	Large, thick, dome shaped muscle creating the round rump of the horse. It originating from the gluteal fascia, the Ilium and the sacroiliac ligaments and inserts into the femur.	Very strong and well developed muscle on dressage and cart horses.
Superficial gluteal muscle	Aids abduction of the hind leg and flexes the pelvis.	Large muscle that originates at the tuba coxae and from the gluteal fascia. It travels underneath the Tensor fascia latae and inserts onto the femur.	
Tensor Fascia Latae	Flexes the pelvis at the point of hip and aids movement of the hind leg forward.	Thick strap muscle that originates at the tuba coxae and inserts around the patella and onto the cranial ridge of the tibia.	Very important muscle when jumping and in collection work.

Biceps Femoris	Part of the hamstring group. Aids the extension of the hind leg, aids abductor and prevents excessive adduction.	Very large superficial muscle that originates high up to the coccygeal / gluteal fascia and to the lateral side of the sacroiliac ligament and travels distally to insert cranially around the patella and to the caudal distal side of the femur.	Very prominent and well developed in horses that jump and race.
Semimembranosis	Part of the Hamstrings group. Plays a large role in the extension of the hind leg and aids adduction of the hind leg.	Long thick muscle that runs medially parallel to Semitendonosis. It originates from the caudal edge of the Sacrosiatic ligament and the ventral side of the tuber ischium. It then inserts onto the medial epicondyle of the femur.	Very prominent in race horses and jumping horses. Very powerful muscle.
Semitendonosis	Part of the Hamstring group. Aids the extension of the hind leg.	Long thick muscle that runs alongside Semimembranosis. It originates from the first 2 coccygeal vertebrae and the ventral side of the tuber ischium and	Very prominent in race horses and jumping horses. Very powerful muscle.

		inserts into the cranial side of the tibia.	
Gastronemius	Flexes the hock and aids extension and abduction of the hind leg.	Small thick muscle that originates from the lateral epicondyle of the femur and the head of the tibia. Inserts as the Achilles tendon.	
Short tail levator muscle	Lifts the tail and aids in lateral movement of the tail when swishing.	Long muscle situated dorsally along the coccygeal vertebrae originating from the sacral vertebrae and gluteal fascia making up the dock of the tail.	
Tail depressor muscle	Lowers the tail, aids lateral movement of the tail when swishing and cranial movement when clamping the tail.	Thick strong muscle that attaches ventrally to the sacral spine at approximately S3 and attaches ventrally along the sacral and coccygeal vertebrae inserting at approximately coccygeal vertebrae 8 – 10.	

Gracilis	Aids the adduction of the hind leg.	Large thick sheet muscle that originates medially to the pubis and inserts onto the medial edge of the tibia and the medial patella ligament.	
Adductor muscle	Adducts the leg turning the femur medially and flexes the hip.	Strong thick strap of muscle that originates from the ventral side of the Pubis and inserts onto the caudal and medial edges of the Femur.	Very important muscle that is used when doing leg yield and half pass.
Rectus Femoris	Aids flexion of the hind leg and flexes the hip.	Thick deep muscle that originates from the Ilium and inserts onto the patella cranially.	One of the four muscles that makes up the Quadriceps along with Vastus Medialis, vastus intermedius and Vastus Lateralis .
Vastus Medialis	Aids the extension of the stifle joint, flexion and adduction of the hind leg.	Strong thick muscle that runs parallel to Rectus Femoris. It originates from the dorsal medial edge of the femur and inserts onto the medial edge of the patella.	One of the Quadriceps muscles.

Sartorius muscle	Flexes the pelvis and sacrum, and aids the flexion of the hind leg.	Long strap muscle that originates at the sacrum and inserts at the patella.	
Psoas minor	Aids flexion of the pelvis.	Small deep muscle that originates from the thorasic vertebrae T16, T17, and T18, and the Lumbar vertebrae L4 and L5; and inserts onto the Ilium.	
Psoas Major	Supports and flexes the pelvis, flexing the hip and aiding abduction of the femur.	Very deep, 'fillet' like muscle. Originates from the ventral surface of the lumbar vertebrae and the lumbosacral junction. It also attaches to the caudal medial upper edge of the last 2 ribs and inserts onto the Minor trochanter of the Femur.	
Internal obdurator muscle	Lines the pelvis and aids lateral rotation of the femur.	Deep sheet muscle that originates from and attaches dorsally to the Pubis, Ilium, Ischium and the sacral wings. It finishes inserting	

		into the trochanter fossa on the caudal side of the femur.	
Iliacus muscle	Stabilises the pelvis but allows for flexion of the hip and lateral rotation of the femur.	Deep seated muscle that is situated under the medial gluteal muscle. It originates from the ventral ridge of the Ilium and inserts as a tendon alongside the psoas major at the minor trochanter of the femur where it intersects with the tendon of the psoas major.	
Sacrosiatic muscle	Supports and flexes the sacrum.	Originates from the ventral surface of the sacrum and the first 3 coccygeal vertebrae, attaching to the tuber sacral and inserts into the pelvis on the dorsal ridge of the Ilium.	
Long digital extensor muscle and tendon	Aids extension of the hind leg forward.	Large muscle that is situated on the cranial lateral side of the hind leg originating from	

		the cranial lateral head of the Tibia and runs down the leg changing into a tendon lying in front of the tarsal bones and continuing down inserting over the pastern and coffin joints.	
Lateral digital extensor muscle	Aids extension and lateral movement of the hind limb.	Large muscle located caudally of the long digital extensor muscle on the lateral side of the hind leg. Originating from the lateral head of the Tibia and fibula and inserting as a tendon to the lateral edge of the pedal bone.	
Deep digital Flexor muscle and tendon	Flexes the hind leg out behind the horse	Large muscle that is located on the lateral caudal side of the hind leg originating from the caudal lateral head of the tibia continues as a tendon that runs superficial of the Suspensory ligament but deeper than the superficial digital	

		flexor tendon and attaches to the pedal bone.	
Achilles Tendon	Extends the hock.	Thick tendon that originates from the gastronemius an inserts at the Calcaneal tuber (point of hock).	
Superficial digital Flexor tendon	Flexes the hock and stretches the hind limb out behind the horse.	Large tendon that runs superficial of the Deep digital flexor over the hock down behind the cannon bone below the fetlock and attaches distally to the long and short pasterns.	
Suspensory ligament	Supports the fetlock and prevents over extension of the joint.	The ligament runs down the hind leg behind the cannon bone between the 2 splint bones and then sections off into 2 branches travelling over the 2 sesamoid bones at the back of the fetlock and continues distally attaching to the lower extensor tendons.	

Equine Bowen Therapy Procedures

Bottom stoppers and Top stoppers

These moves are used to start every treatment as they prepare the horses body by segmenting the nervous system and energy into 3 areas – the hind quarters, the main trunk of the body, and the front end (shoulders, head and neck). The horses body is then ready to undergo the rest of the treatment and is able to relax and begin responding immediately and effectively.

The Bottom stoppers are performed over the lumber area either side of the horse's spine centred between the two points of hips, over Longissimus dorsi.

Firstly the therapist will locate the point of hip on both sides and create an imaginary line between the two to the spine in the centre. Two medial Bowen moves are then carried out either side of the spine over the Longissimus dorsi muscle; the first 2 Bowen moves are made slightly cranially of points of hips and the next 2 moves are made approximately 2 inches caudally of the previous moves . These moves temporarily divide up the horses nervous system and disconnects the energy in the hind quarters from the rest of the body. These moves over Longissimus dorsi will also have some effect on the surrounding muscles such as sacrospinalis ligament, psoas major and psoas minor.

Next the Top stoppers are performed across the withers of the horse. Again two medial Bowen moves are required either side of the spine to release the trapezius muscle and separate the shoulders, forelimbs, head and neck from the rest of the body.

The Therapist needs to visualise a line through the very middle of the withers separating the withers into 2 sections. The medial Bowen moves are then made approximately 2 inches lower than the spine, 2 moves each side, and one move is made in each visualised section spaced approximately 2 inches apart. The 2 Bowen moves over the thoracic trapezius are made first followed by the next 2 Bowen moves over the cervical trapezius. These moves may also effect the surrounding muscles such as the rhomboids that sit deeper underneath the trapezius, attaching to the top of the Nucheal ligament and scapular.

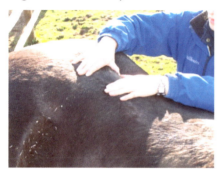 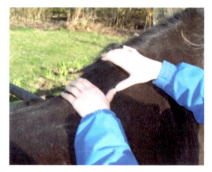

Above: 1st of the Bottom Stoppers on the nearside and 1st of the Top stoppers on the offside

The above moves are then usually followed by moves over the Tensor Fascia Latae; a deep significant muscle situated in the pelvis, and then a 2 minute break to allow the horses body to react accordingly.

Hamstring Procedure

The hamstrings running down the back of the horses hind legs are separated into 2 muscles that run side by side; semi membranosus and semi tendinosus. These muscles are highly powerful and the condition of these muscles has a massive effect of the horses performance and ability.

The therapist will firstly treat the medial of the 2 muscles, semi membranosus, and make approximately 4 evenly spaced lateral Bowen moves along the length of the muscle beginning at the top by the top of the dock, and finishing at the base of the muscle where it semi membranosus meets gracilis.

The therapist then returns to the top of semi tendinosus and locates the separation between the 2 hamstring muscles. 4 evenly spaced, approximately 6 inches apart, lateral Bowen moves are then carried out along semi tendinosus. As the muscle narrows below the gastronemius muscle, it then becomes tendon, known as Achilles tendon. Another 2 lateral Bowen moves are made over the tendon, one at the head of the tendon and one just above the hock.

This procedure is usually followed by moves made over gastronemius, this muscle equates to the calf muscles in a human, followed by a 2 minute break.

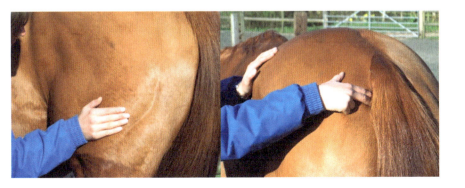

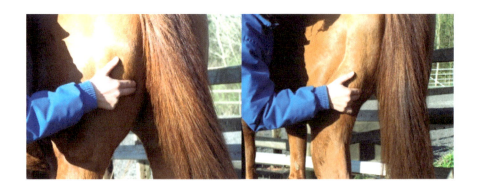
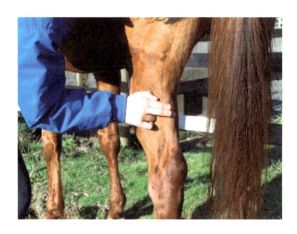

Opening the back

Before this procedure is performed the bottom and top stoppers need to be repeated to keep the body divided into the 3 sections.

After the therapist has done the top stoppers they then begin to open the back by making medial moves, 2 inches apart, along the length of the Longissimus dorsi, starting 2 inches cranially of the last bottom stopper and finishing before the first top stopper. The therapist should note any areas of pain or discomfort along this muscle all it is the main muscle that supports the saddle and rider. An ill fitting saddle can have a damaging effect on this muscle. By opening the back you release Longissimus dorsi and the surrounding muscles allowing the horse to move more freely through its back both longitudinally and laterally.

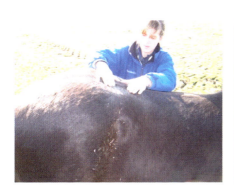
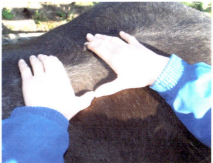
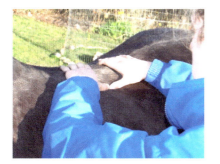
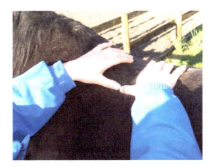

Respiratory procedure

This procedure is fantastic for horses with any breathing issues and horses that find it hard to bend through their bodies. The therapist and handler must both be aware of the horse's behaviour during this procedure as some horses can be sensitive under their belly and around the edge of the ribcage.

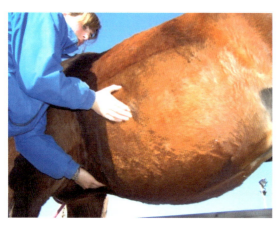

Firstly the therapist needs to locate the centre of the sternum and, when starting on the left side, place the pads of their fingers on their left hand there as a holding point. Then with their fingers on their right hand the therapist needs to find the edge of the ribcage and make 3 – 5 Bowen moves along the edge of the ribcage, cranially to caudally (front to back), challenging the muscles directly underneath the ribcage and then allowing the muscles and the edge of the ribs to roll underneath their fingers. This releases any tension along the ribcage and is repeated on the other side this time with the therapist placing their right hand in the centre of the sternum and using the left hand to create the moves.

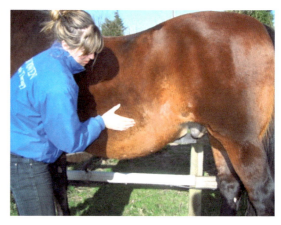

The therapist then removes their hand from the centre of the sternum and makes 3 moves just caudally of the sternum along the centre line of the body approximately an inch apart one behind the other. This can help to move any unwanted fluid that has been left in the lungs which can build up in

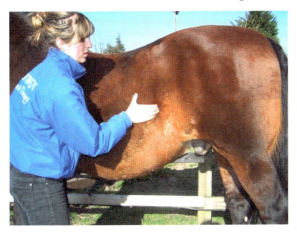

horses with allergies, respiratory problems, or horses that are kept in dusty conditions or keep in the stable for large amounts of time. Horses usually give a good sigh or a big deep breath after this procedure as the rib cage, the lungs and the diaphragm have all been relaxed and released.

This procedure can be followed by a wither lift stretch (see page ?), which can be especially beneficial for horses that are tight or stiff in the back.

Shoulder procedure (Rhomboids, trapezius and Subclavius)

This procedure is usually preceded by moves over and around the patella, followed by a repeat of the top stoppers to isolate the front section of the horse or pony.

Horses that are very upright in the shoulders, highly strung, nervous, stressy, or been through a trauma tend to be tight or hold a lot of tension in and around their shoulders especially through Subclavius, also known as Deep Cranial Pectoralis (DCP).

Firstly the therapist will begin by making moves around the head of the scapular starting at the upper caudal edge of the scapular, these moves are releasing and stimulating the rhomboids and trapezius muscles.

The therapist uses their thumbs, tip to tip, moving the skin slack caudally challenging the muscle and then moving cranially over the muscle following the edge of the scapular. The therapist then lifts their thumbs above where they finished the last move releasing the skin and then replaces their thumbs back where they were and repeats the move again. The therapist my need to repeat the move 5 to 12 times depending on the size of the horse or pony and also the availability of skin slack depending on how taught the skin is.

This completes the first half of the shoulder procedure which is carried out firstly on the left side and then the right side of the horse, before returning to the left side to begin the second half of the procedure.

The second half of the procedure works on releasing Subclavius, also known as Deep Cranial Pectoralis (DCP), and opening up the shoulders. Subclavius is located just in front of the scapular, it originates deep in the horse at the front of the sternum and inserts along the front edge of the scapular.

To locate Subclavius the therapist needs to stand next to the horse facing forwards and quietly place their hand on the horse's nose, persuading the horse to bend its head and neck round toward the therapist. This takes some of the tension out of the muscle and allows the therapist to place their hand nearest the horse over the top of the muscle, approximately half way down the front of the scapular and use their fingers to tuck under the front edge of the scapular. The therapist will then challenge the muscle and then release it allowing the muscle to roll back underneath their fingers.

If the horse is tight through its shoulders and/or neck then they may find this difficult and may resist or pull away from the therapist. If this happens the therapist must be patient and keep quietly encouraging the horse to cooperate until they relax and become submissive. The therapist will always work within the horses limitations as this keeps the horse relaxed and in the best state for optimum results. If the horse is stiff or tight in this area then you can release the horses head after the first move and then get the horse back in position ready for the second move.

The therapist then makes a second move ¾'s of the way down the front of the scapular. Again with the horses head bent around toward the therapist, the therapist tucks there hand under the front edge of the scapular and challenges the muscle. If the horse is relatively relaxed and free through its shoulder when the therapist challenges the muscle it is possible for Subclavius to be lifted up and out in front of the scapular. Again the muscle is released and allowed to roll back under the therapists hands, and the therapist can now let go of the horses head also. The therapist will then repeat these moves on the right side of the horse followed by a 2 minute break.

Horses tend to have considerable reactions after this procedure, and in my opinion it is a very important and telling muscular and neurological release that occurs in the horse's body. The horse's owner, rider or groom can then continue to improve the horse's flexibility and movement through the horses shoulders by doing daily stretches with the horse, both static and dynamic, such as leg yielding when ridden and carrot stretches after exercise (see pages ? - ?).

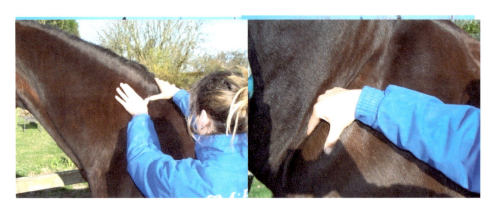

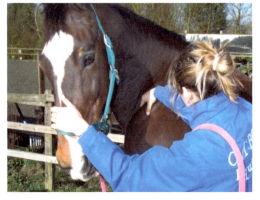

Tempra Mandibular Joint (TMJ) Procedure

The Tempra Mandibular joints are the hinge joints of the horses jaw and are located either side of the horses head set below the ears, but distal and caudal the horse's eyes. The positioning of the TMJ usually correlates with the position of the pelvis, therefore if the horses jaw is out of line a good dentist should refer you to an Equine Therapist where it is Bowen, McTimony, and Acupuncture etc.

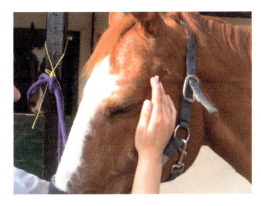

1) Standing to the front of the horses head locate the Tempra Mandibular joints on either side of the horses head using your middle fingers. Hold your fingers there for a minimum of 5 seconds, this makes the horses brain and nervous system aware of these joints. Notice an differences between the left and right side such as tension, stiffness, the joints position on the horses head especially height.

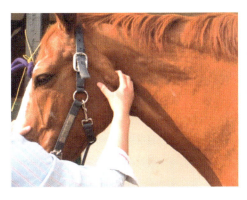

2) Using the pads of your fingers place them along the ? muscle just below the wing of atlas behind the jaw and draw the skin slack medially in towards the horse. Apply eye ball pressure and challenge the

muscle; when the horse is relax the ? muscle should 'pop out' along the ridge of the jaw. Slowly release the muscle allowing it to move underneath your fingers. Repeat on the opposite side.

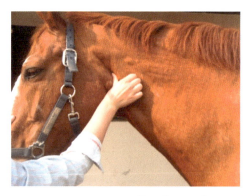

3) Approximately 3inches below the wing of atlas along sternoclediomastoid place the pad of your thumb and draw skin slack towards the horses head. Apply eye ball pressure then make move ventrally along the muscle. remove your thumb then replace it 1 inch below the previous move and repeat the same move again. Repeat moves on the opposite side.

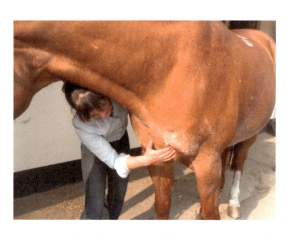

4) Staying on the offside, using your right hand on the near side of the horses chest and with the bulb of your hand (base of your palm) draw the horses skin slack medially to the horses sternum. Apply eye ball pressure and slowly move laterally across the horses chest. Position yourself on the horses nearside and repeat the move with your left hand on the offside of the horses chest.

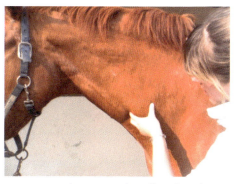

5) Using the pads of your index and middle fingers on your left hand, starting at the base of braceociphalic muscle, draw skinslack medially in towards the horse around the muscle. Apply eyeball pressure and gently release the muscle allowing it to roll underneath you fingers. Repeat this move another 3 -4 times along the length of braceociphalic making sure they are evenly spaced. Notice any differences through the muscle as you work up towards the head.

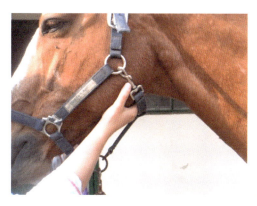

6) Position yourself in front of the horse. Cup both of your hands with the backs of your fingers touching in behind the horses jaw between the two jaw bones and gently apply pressure in the centre using your finger tips. Steadily move your fingers slightly right and left, essentially creating a wiggling action for minimum of 5 seconds. This creates a vibration to release the muscles surrounding the hyoid bones which are connected to the tongue, ears and eyes. This is a sensitive area especially if the horse is tight or may have been ear or tongue twitched / tied.

7) Starting on the horses nearside of their face, place your index and middle fingers just below the Tempra Mandibular joint. Imagine a line between the Tempra mandibular joint and the corner of horse's mouth. Make 4 or 5 evenly spaced moves down along the

massater muscle towards the corner of the horse's mouth by drawing the skin slack up, apply eye ball pressure and move directly downwards. Remove your fingers and replace them below the previous move and repeat till you reach the horse's mouth. Repeat the moves on the other side of the horses face. Notice the horses reactions after you have performed these moves.

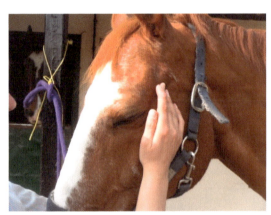

8) Stay positioned in front of the horses head. Place your middle fingers either side of the horses head on the Tempra mandibular joint. Keeping both fingers in place, start on the horses nearside draw the skin slack upwards, apply eye ball pressure and then move directly downwards. Without lifting your finger off return your finger back to its original position then draw the skin slack cranially towards yourself, apply eye ball pressure then move directly caudally. Again without removing your finger return it to its original position. Keeping both fingers still in place repeat the moves from the nearside on the horses offside using your left hand. Once these moves are complete remove both hands at the same time and notice the horses reactions.

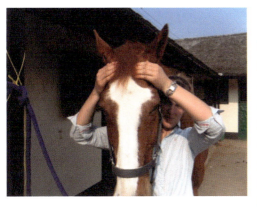

9) Reposition yourself beside the horses neck facing in the same direction as the horse. Stretch your right arm underneath the horses head and neck and using both hands place the pads of your fingers along the medial edges of the fatty pads situated below the horses ears. Starting with your left hand draw the horses skin slack medially, apply eyeball pressure the make the move laterally. Repeat this move on the right hand side using your right hand. Notice the horses response after this move as it can be a big release for some horses.

Stretching the horse

In relation to Equine Bowen Therapy, stretching is a great way for the horses' owner to maximise the effectiveness of the treatment, therefore prolonging the benefit the horse receives. A good therapist is able to advise a client on how to stretch their horse correctly and in the most effective way that is specific to the horses needs. Regular stretching will help to maintain and improve the horses range of movement, flexibility, and suppleness to improve the horses performance and also minimise muscle fatigue and reduce the risk of injury by minimising the tension through the muscles and tendons, in turn reducing stress on the horses joints. In terms of performance this could mean a horse is more expressive through its paces scoring higher marks in dressage, a racehorse could gain a longer stride length due to more flexibility through its pelvis and hamstrings increasing the chance of winning, a show jumper / event horse could become more agile over a fence and turning round a course due to increased flexibility and suppleness through its body as could a polo pony increase its acceleration speed and ability to turn.

Stretching is easy and can be incorporated into the a horses daily routine with minimal fuss and, depending on the horse, a significant improvement in the horse can be noticed within a matter of a couple of weeks. There are three different types of stretching which all have the potential to help any horse; passive stretching, active stretching and autonomic reflex reaction stretching. Bearing this in mind there are also some rules to stretching which make sure stretching is done in the most safe and effective way.

Rules of stretching

- A horse / pony must only be stretched after the muscles have been warmed up, for example after the horse has been ridden or walked out in hand for at least approximately 15 minutes.
- Always ensure that you and the horse are stood on level ground and on a non slip surface.
- If needed have another person to hold the horse whilst you do the stretches, If not make sure there is somewhere to tie up the horse correctly using a quick release knot.
- Always put the safety of you and other people around the horse first.
- Make sure the area you are stretching in has sufficient light to work safely and has more than enough room for you to work around the horse. Also ensure there is plenty of head room in case the horse throws its head in the air.
- Before you carry out any stretch on the fore or hind limbs make sure you always start with a relaxation stretch to ensure that the joints are warmed up and prepared for the stretch.
- Make sure the horse is stood square before stretching so the horse is able to balance.
- It is wise to run your hands all over the horses body before starting so you are aware of any sensitive areas the horse may have.
- Always stretch the horse within its capabilities, so do not over stretch.

- Hold each stretch for a minimum of 5 seconds and build it up so you are able to hold the horse in a stretch for 15 seconds.
- Always place the horses legs back on the floor after a stretch, never just let go and drop them. Occasionally a horse will snatch its leg back; if this happens just make sure you are not over stretching. Keep as much control of the horses limbs as possible.
- When you stretch a horse make sure you hold the correct posture as shown to protect your own back and make sure you and anybody else helping has the correct clothing and footwear on. When using both hands to hold a stretch make sure you overlap your hands and do not interlock your fingers.

Forms of stretching

Passive stretching

Passive stretching, also known as static stretching, is done with the horse held in hand so the handler cares out the stretches on the ground. These stretches are always done immediately after the horse has worked and the muscles are warmed up. It is most beneficial to have a stretch programme worked out that you can do straight after you have ridden the horse as this is a great way to combine stretching, spending time bonding with the horse and given them a well deserved carrot or equivalent treat.

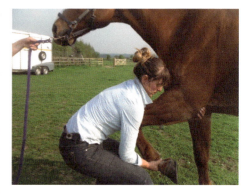

Active stretching

Active stretching is also known as dynamic stretching and is done whilst riding the horse. The main thing to remember when doing lateral stretches such as those based on leg yielding is that it does not have to look like a correct dressage movement with the horse on the bit; it is just a case of getting the horse moving around in a relaxed way to stretch specific areas of the horses body to improve the performance and wellbeing of horse in the best and most effective way possible. I would advise that you ask your instructor or equine therapist to explain to you how to carry out the different lateral movements that you require to help stretch your horse whilst riding. I would always start lateral stretching in walk to establish the control of the stretch and it is easier to explain it to a horse that isn't used to doing lateral work or a horse that is laterally stiff.

Autonomic reflex reaction stretching

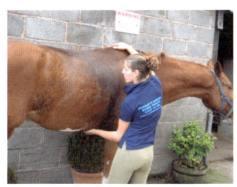

Autonomic reflex reaction stretching works on getting the horse to stretch areas of its own body by stimulating a specific reflex and as they react they stretch the opposing area. All the Autonomic stretches in this book are all performed with the horse in hand.

Stretches

When you are stretching a horse the most important safety factor to consider is yourself and your own posture. It is important when stretching that you adopt the Basic positional posture for a stretch to protect your back and minimise any stresses being put on you through weight bearing.

In the following text your outer hand, arm, or leg is the side furthest away from the horse and your inner hand, arm, or leg is the side nearest the horse.

Stand next to the horse, usually facing towards the back of the horse, and spread your legs apart with your outer leg forward and your inner leg back; this gives you better balance and mobility when stretching. When holding the horse's leg, make sure you bend your knees and if possible always have you outer elbow resting on your outer knee to support your back.

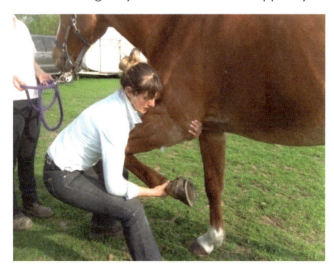

Above – demonstrating the basic positional posture being used during a tricep stretch allowing the therapist to stretch the horse effectively and safely.

Passive Stretches for the forehand.

Relaxation stretch.

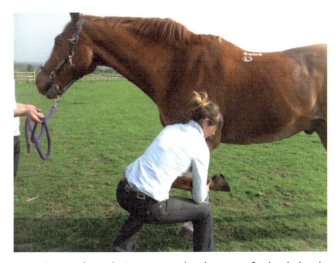

Adopt the 'Basic positional posture for a leg stretch'. Ask the horse to bend at his knee or hock and pick up its hoof using your inner hand. Support the horses fetlock by holding it with both hands (do not interlock your fingers), bend your own knees and place your outer elbow on your outer knee to support your back. Begin by slowly moving the horses leg forwards and backwards shifting your own weight through your body to do so. Repeat this 4 or 5 times then bring the horses leg back to the centre where you began. Next rotate the horses hoof slowly in circles, firstly clockwise then anti clockwise, doing 4 to 5 rotations each way. Repeat this on both front legs and hind legs noting any differences. Make sure you place the horses hoof back down after the stretch or alternatively go straight into another foreleg or hind leg stretch.

Tricep stretch

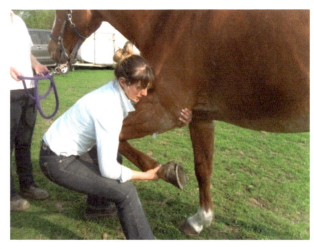

Either continue from the relaxation stretch or adopt the 'basic positional posture for a leg stretch' and ask the horse to bend its knee and pick its hoof up. Hold the fetlock with your outer hand and take your inner hand and stroke the inside of the horses forearm and place the palm of your inner hand on the inside just above the horses elbow. Ask the horse to stretch forward and down slightly shifting your body weight to carry the horses leg. Hold the stretch for 5 – 15 seconds at a time, this stretch can be repeated if the horse is willing; note if the horse is able to stretch further or hold the stretch for longer if it is repeated.

Forearm Stretch (Elbow flexor / Carpi extensor)

Adopt the 'basic positional posture for a leg stretch' standing slightly in front of the horses shoulder and ask the horse to bend its knee and pick up its hoof. Rest your inner shoulder up against the horses forearm positioning your inner arm on the inside of the horse's leg using your inner hand and outer hand to support the fetlock joint, or alternatively if it's more comfortable or the horse is resistant you can use one hand to support the fetlock and the other on the front of the horses knee to help stabilise the stretch. Gently shifting your body weight forward, slowly stretch the horse's leg back underneath its self and slightly downward. Hold the stretch for 5 – 15 seconds and then bring the horses leg back to its original position and place its hoof back on the ground. Repeat this stretch on both front legs.

Extending Girth stretch

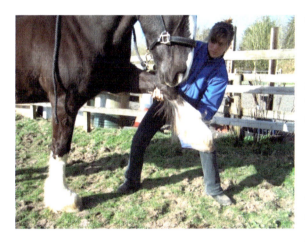

Take on the 'Basic positional posture for a leg stretch' this time facing towards the front of the horse. Ask the horse to bend its knee and lift it forward using your inner hand and forearm to support underneath the horses knee. Use your Outer hand to support the fetlock ensuring that you rest your outer elbow on your outer leg. Now by shifting you body weight and position forward, ask the horse to stretch its leg forwards and down, keeping a slight bend in the horses knee joint. Hold the stretch for 5 – 15 seconds, and then take the horse's leg back to its original position and place its hoof back down on the ground. Repeat this stretch on both front legs noting any differences: If one leg is significantly stiffer or less flexible than the other it is worth repeating this stretch on the worse side once more a two minutes after you did it the first time.

Lateral shoulder stretch

Adopt the 'basic positional posture for leg stretch' next to the horses shoulder and ask the horse to bend its knee and pick up its hoof. Use your outer hand to hold 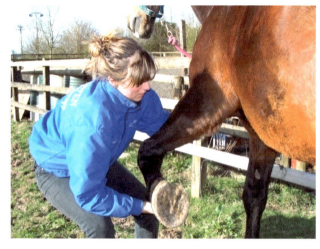 and support the front of the fetlock joint and position your inner hand high up on the inside of the horses forearm keeping the horses leg relatively straight always ensuring a slight bend at the knee to protect the horses joints. Make sure you place your outer elbow on your outer leg to protect your back and joints as well. Using your inner hand to push and your outer hand to guide, move your body weight laterally and ask the horse to stretch its leg directly outwards (laterally) and slightly down. Hold the stretch for 5 – 15 seconds and then bring the horse's leg back to its original position and place its hoof on the ground. Repeat this stretch on both front legs.

NB – This stretch is great for horses that are built very upright or tight in the shoulder, horses that find lateral work difficult.

Medial shoulder and forearm stretch

Once again adopt the 'basic positional posture for a leg stretch' standing next to the horses shoulder and ask the horse to bend its knee and pick its hoof up. Use your inner hand to support the horses fetlock and put your outer hand against the outer edge of the horses elbow. Pushing with your outer hand ask the horse to stretch its forearm underneath itself towards the midline of the horse's body. Hold the stretch for 5 – 15 second then bring the horses leg back to its

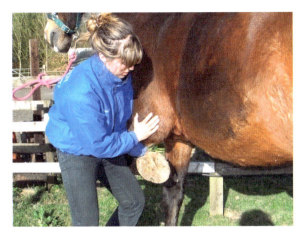

original position and place its hoof back on the floor. Repeat this stretch on both front legs.

NB – This stretch stretches all the muscles on the outside of the forearm and the outside of the scapular all the way from the upper edge of the scapular. This stretch is fantastic for horses that find it hard to extend their strides in front, horses that find lateral work difficult, horses that are built upright and narrow in the shoulder, horses that find it hard to change direction quickly and on acute angles and / or horses that find it hard or are slow to pick up their forelegs over a fence.

Passive stretches for the main trunk of the body

Wither lift (autonomic reflex reaction stretch)

Be aware that some horses may be sensitive under their ribcage around their girth area and so may react by kicking out and biting.

Firstly you need to locate the centre of the horse's sternum using your finger tips.

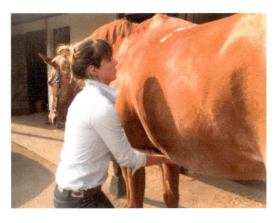

Place your hands side by side and scoop your hand so the pads of your fingertips are positioned in the centre of the horses sternum and then gently apply pressure upwards. Watch as the horses neck lowers and the back lifts up away from your hands. If the horse is stiff through his back then he may only be able to lift a little to begin with. If the horse resists lifting his back then wiggle your fingers to encourage the lift but make sure you force the stretch as this can aggravate the horse and cause him to tense up.

Tail Stretch

This stretch aims to help release the muscles across the top of the back especially the supra spinous ligament and those that closely lye alongside the spinous processes.

This stretch involves standing directly behind the horse so must only be performed if the therapist or person performing the stretch is confident that the horse will not kick out with its hind legs.

Firstly have the horse standing square with all 4 legs so the stretch is carried out evenly through the horses body. The person carrying out the stretch must position themselves in a stance with one foot half a stride forward of the other to retain balance and control during the stretch. Using both hands lift and hold the horses tail part way down the dock, then shift your body weight back whilst holding on to the horses dock and gently take a pull. Most horses will lean forward into the stretch lowering their head and neck forward and down so make sure you control and maintain a stable stretch so the horse doesn't all forward and jar themselves. Watch how the horses back lifts and stretches over the top of the pelvis, through the back and into the neck. Also be aware if the horse is uncomfortable or tighter on one side of the back they may swing or lean one way with their quarters or will move a hind leg either underneath themselves or out behind them to lessen the stretch over a particular area. If you are able to isolate a tighter area you can follow the tail stretch with a carrot stretch to help release that particular area and then go back and do another tail stretch and see the difference from the first tail stretch. Hold the stretch for 5 – 15 seconds then release the horses tail slowly as most horses will be leaning against the stretch and have their body weight forward. Notice how the horse reacts after the stretch has released.

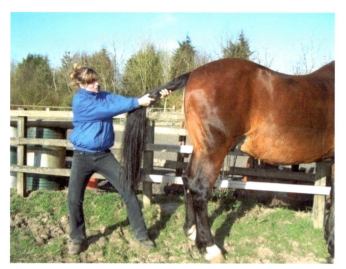

Above - demonstrating the extent of the stretch over the horses back during a tail stretch with the horse stood square to get an even stretch.

Passive stretching for the whole body head and neck

Carrot stretches

These stretches are great fun for both horse and handler, and are a fantastic way to reward your horse after exercise and stretch at the same time.

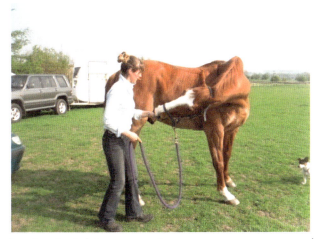

The first thing to remember is to get a large supply of carrots and keep them in a clean and dry box outside the horses stable. To begin stretching, ensuring you are on a non slip surface and the horses muscles have been warmed up, get a carrot and show it to the horse. When the horse is interested in the carrot bring the carrot back towards the horses hind quarters about half way up the height of the horse and the horse should follow with their head and neck. This stretches the muscles on the other side of the horses body. Make sure the horse is stretching as far as they are able to then hold it for 5 seconds before giving the carrot to the horse and allowing them to relax back their head and neck. Repeat this on both sides. Next take another carrot back towards the horses hind quarters this time lower down about a quarter of the way p the horses height; notice if the horse find this harder or easier than the previous stretch, repeat on both sides. For the third side stretch take a carrot towards the horses hind quarters holding it three quarters of the way up the horses height; again notice if this is a harder or easier stretch for the horse than the previous stretches. If you want to see how the muscles stretch then get somebody else to perform the stretches and then you can stand on the opposite side and observe.

You can also stretch the horses topline and over the back using carrot stretches. For this stretch you need to make sure the horse si stood square, then get a carrot and bring it down in between the horses front legs getting the horse to bring their head and neck down between its knees and as far back as the horse can go. Getting the horse to reach for the carrot at varied interval heights stretches all the different muscle groups on the opposite side.

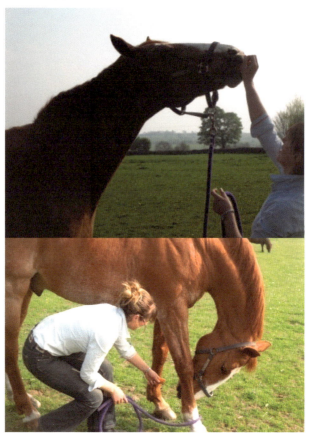

Passive Stretching for the hind quarters

Before performing any of the following hind leg stretches you must firstly loosen up the joints of the hind leg you wish to stretch by carrying out a relaxation stretch as shown in Passive stretches for the forehand. Be conscious that horses that suffer from wobblers syndrome or a similar neurological condition my either find hind leg stretches difficult or they may not be able to perform them at all.

Hamstring stretch

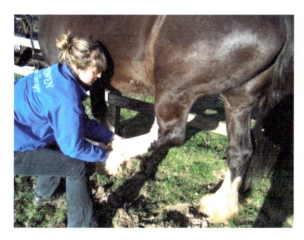

Either continue from the relaxation stretch or adopt the 'basic positional posture for a leg stretch' and ask the horse to lift up its hind leg. Move yourself in position cranially, back towards the horses head, and place your hands one on top of the other cupping and supporting the fetlock joint. Now by moving your body weight back ask the horse to stretch its hind leg forward under its body and down towards the ground. Make sure to ask the horse to stretch gently and slowly. Hold the stretch for 5 – 15 second and then either place the horses hoof down directly below the stretch, this is a good way of measuring the horses progress when stretching over a period of weeks or months, or return the horses leg to its original position. Be aware that if the horse is uncomfortable then they may snatch their leg back so the person stretching needs to start again making sure they are not forcing the horse to stretch more than is capable.

Quadriceps stretch

Horses with stifle injuries or who have had recent treatment to the stifle MUST NOT be asked to perform this stretch.

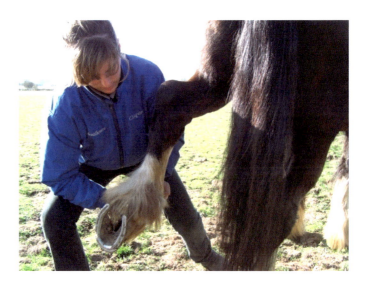

Continuing from the relaxation stretch maintaining the basic positional posture with both hands overlapping under the horses fetlock supporting the joint. Gently move your body weight forward onto your front leg and guide the horses leg to stretch out behind them. Be aware that the horse may snatch their leg back underneath themselves so make sure your leg is not in the way and perform the stretch gradually. Hold the stretch for 5 – 15 seconds then slowly guide the horses leg back to its original position and either replace on to the ground or go into another stretch. This stretch is especially good for horses that are tight / stiff in their pelvis, jumping horses, and race horses. It can also help your horse be more comfortable and therefore easier to handle when being shod by the farrier.

Abductor and medial gluteal stretch

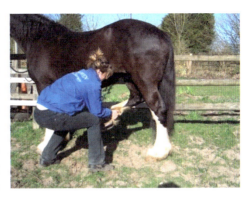

After placing the horses hoof back to the ground after the relaxation stretch or other previous stretches, go around to the opposite side of the horse, reach underneath the horses hind quarters and ask them to pick up the same leg again. Some horses may be confused so get somebody to help by lifting up the horse's leg and then pass it over to you. Adopt the basic positional posture with both your hands overlapping underneath the horses fetlock joint. Slowly guide the horses leg slightly forward and underneath itself across in front of its other hind leg. Remember to stretch gradually and within the horses comfort zone as they may feel slightly off balance during this stretch. Hold the stretch for 5 – 15 seconds then steadily allow the horse's leg to go back to its original resting position. Horses that are lateral stiff behind can really benefit from this stretch.

Adductor stretch

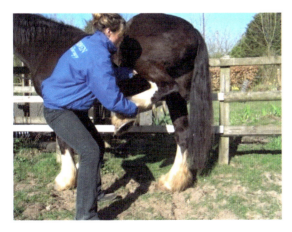

When performing this stretch it generally isn't possible to rest your outer elbow on your outer leg so only perform this stretch if you are confident to do so and do not suffer from serve bad back. Continue from a relaxation stretch or ask the horse to lift up its hind leg. Standing to the side of the horse adopt the same leg stance from the basic positional posture, place your outer hand behind and under the fetlock joint and place the palm of your inner hand confidently inside the top of the horses just below the stifle.

Gradually ask the horse to stretch its leg laterally away from its body opening up the gap between its hind legs. Some horses my feel slightly off balance so it is important to do this stretch slowly. Hold the stretch for 5 – 15 seconds then gently replace the horses leg back to its original resting place. Horses that are either base narrow or more straight legged in their confirmation 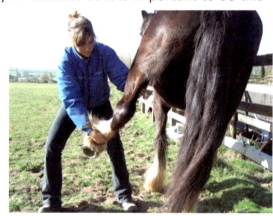 behind, display pelvic stiffness or unusual hind leg action may benefit from this stretch.

USEFUL LINKS

Charlotte Maguire cert ECBS, RFCES
T: 07825180980
E: bowen@cmbowen.co.uk
W: www.cmbowen.co.uk

European College of Bowen Studies
T: 01373832340
E: info@thebowentechnique.com
W: www.thebowentechnique.com

Rose Farm College of Equine Studies
T: 01278 723429
E: lotty.merry@rosefarmequine.co.uk
W: www.rosefarmequine.co.uk

W.E.S. Garrett Saddlers
T: 01934 742367
A: WES Garrett Saddlers, Back Lane, Draycott
 Somerset, BS27 3TS

Pro-Motion Equine
T: 07789265683
E: info@promotionequine.co.uk
W: www.promotionequine.co.uk

Institution of Applied Equine Podiatry (IAEP)
T: 800-351-2741
E: baremysole@yahoo.com
W: www.appliedequinepodiatory.org

Farrier Register
T: 01733319911
E: frc@farrier-reg.gov.uk
W: www.farrier-reg.gov.uk

British Horse Society
T: 08448481666
W: www.bhs.org.uk

Harry Meade - GB Event rider
E: info@harrymeade.co.uk
W: www.harrymeade.co.uk

Burcott Riding Centre
T: 01749673145
W: www.burcottriddingcentre.co.uk

British Association of Equine Dental Technicians
T: 07500 462669
W: www.baedt.com

Equidentist – Charlotte white
T: 07795141845
E: charlotte@equidentist.co.uk
W: www.equidentist.co.uk

Rosamund Green Farm – Millie Dumas (GB event rider), Proven and potential event horses for sale, cross country course, Livery and schooling.
T: 01749343384
E: r.k.dumas@btinternet.com
W: www.rosamundgreenfarm.co.uk

Horse 'n' Art - Julia Davie Equestrian Artist
T: 01749 870264
E: barry.davie@virgin.net

Printed in Great Britain
by Amazon